Frozen Section Library: Appendix, Colon, and Anus

For further volumes:
http://www.springer.com/series/7869

Frozen Section Library: Appendix, Colon, and Anus

Nicole C. Panarelli, MD
Weill Medical College of Cornell University, New York, NY

Rhonda K. Yantiss, MD
Weill Medical College of Cornell University, New York, NY

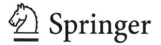 Springer

Nicole C. Panarelli
Weill Medical College
Cornell University
525 East 68th St.
10065 New York, NY
USA
nip9020@nyp.org

Rhonda K. Yantiss
Weill Medical College
Cornell University
525 East 68th St.
10065 New York, NY
USA
rhy2001@med.cornell.edu

ISSN 1868-4157　　　　　e-ISSN 1868-4165
ISBN 978-1-4419-6583-7　　e-ISBN 978-1-4419-6584-4
DOI 10.1007/978-1-4419-6584-4
Springer New York Dordrecht Heidelberg London

Library of Congress Control Number: 2010930654

Printed on acid-free paper

Springer is part of Springer Science+Business Media (www.springer.com)

Preface

Despite many recent advances in ancillary techniques, intraoperative pathology consultation remains one of the most diagnostically and technically challenging areas of surgical pathology. Frozen sections are usually performed while the patient is under general anesthesia and often form the basis for making immediate treatment decisions. Therefore, pathologists must render a diagnosis quickly, despite the pitfalls and artifacts associated with frozen section preparation. Unfortunately, most standard pathology textbooks largely ignore the topic of frozen section, and the value of gross examination of surgical resection specimens is no longer emphasized in many training programs.

Frozen Section Library: Appendix, Colon, and Anus is a volume in the *Frozen Section Library Series*. The book is divided into seven chapters, each of which discusses the clinical context in which a frozen section consultation may be requested. The chapters emphasize gross characteristics of disorders of the lower gastrointestinal tract, address common questions pathologists must answer during frozen section examination, and discuss pitfalls encountered during frozen section analysis. Recommendations regarding specimen handling are also provided.

We hope that this monograph satisfies the need for practical guidelines for the handling and interpretation of resection specimens and facilitates communications between surgical pathologists and our surgical colleagues.

New York, NY

Nicole C. Panarelli
Rhonda K. Yantiss

Series Preface

For over 100 years, the frozen section has been utilized as a tool for the rapid diagnosis of specimens while a patient is undergoing surgery, usually under general anesthesia, as a basis for making immediate treatment decisions. Frozen section diagnosis is often a challenge for the pathologist who must render a diagnosis that has crucial import for the patient in a minimal amount of time. In addition to the need for rapid recall of differential diagnoses, there are many pitfalls and artifacts that add to the risk of frozen section diagnosis that are not present with permanent sections of fully processed tissues that can be examined in a more leisurely fashion. Despite the century-long utilization of frozen sections, most standard pathology textbooks, both general and subspecialty, largely ignore the topic of frozen sections. Few textbooks have ever focused exclusively on frozen section diagnosis and those textbooks that have done so are now out-of-date and have limited illustrations.

The *Frozen Section Library Series* is meant to provide convenient, user-friendly handbooks for each organ system to expedite use in the rushed frozen section situation. These books are small and light-weight, copiously color illustrated with images of actual frozen sections, highlighting pitfalls, artifacts, and differential diagnosis. The advantages of a series of organ-specific handbooks, in addition to the ease-of-use and manageable size, are that (1) a series allows more comprehensive coverage of more diagnoses, both common and rare, than a single volume that tries to highlight a limited number of diagnoses for each organ and (2) a series allows more detailed insight by permitting experienced authorities to emphasize the peculiarities of frozen section for each organ system.

As a handbook for practicing pathologists, these books will be indispensable aids to diagnosis and avoiding dangers in one of the most challenging situations that pathologists encounter. Rapid consideration of differential diagnoses and how to avoid traps caused by frozen section artifacts are emphasized in these handbooks. A series of concise, easy-to-use, well-illustrated handbooks alleviates the often frustrating and time-consuming, sometimes futile, process of searching through bulky textbooks that are unlikely to illustrate or discuss pathologic diagnoses from the perspective of frozen sections in the first place. Tables and charts will provide guidance for differential diagnosis of various histologic patterns. Touch preparations, which are used for some organs such as central nervous system or thyroid more often than others, are appropriately emphasized and illustrated according to the need for each specific organ.

This series is meant to benefit practicing surgical pathologists, both community and academic, and pathology residents and fellows; and also to provide valuable perspectives to surgeons, surgery residents, and fellows who must rely on frozen section diagnosis by their pathologists. Most of all, we hope that this series contributes to the improved care of patients who rely on the frozen section to help guide their treatment.

Philip T. Cagle
Series Editor

Contents

Chapter 1
Intraoperative Evaluation of Colorectal Specimens Containing Cancer

Abstract Intraoperative assessment of colon cancer resection specimens may influence immediate surgical management. Indications for evaluation include determining the depth of invasion, presence of serosal penetration, status of margins, and intactness of the mesorectum, when present. Pathologists may also be asked to identify residual carcinoma in neoadjuvantly treated patients, or document the presence of other lesions, such as adenomas, polypectomy sites, or underlying colitis. Estimating the depth of invasion into the colonic wall is best achieved by macroscopic examination in combination with frozen section analysis, whereas detecting serosal involvement may require touch or scrape preparations of the serosal surface. Assessment of margins is most challenging in rectal specimens, particularly when patients have received neoadjuvant therapy.

Keywords Colonic adenocarcinoma · Serosa · Margins · Mesorectum · Neoadjuvant therapy

Introduction

Colorectal carcinoma is the most common carcinoma of the gastrointestinal tract, and more than 150,000 cases are diagnosed in the United States each year [1]. Surgical excision remains the mainstay of therapy, and pathologic assessment of resection specimens is critically important to the subsequent management of the patient. Pathologic evaluation is necessary to determine the extent of disease, which is the single most powerful predictor of outcome among colorectal cancer patients, and use of the TNM staging system is now standard practice in the United States [2]. Intraoperative assessment of cancer resection specimens may influence immediate management, and indications for evaluation include determining (1) the depth of invasion, (2) presence of serosal penetration, (3) status of margins, and (4) intactness of the mesorectum; identifying residual carcinoma in neoadjuvantly treated patients; and documenting the presence of other lesions, such as polyps, dysplasia in chronic colitis, and tattoos from prior procedures.

Assessing Local Extent of Colorectal Carcinoma

The designations for pathologic tumor stage (pT) describe the deepest point of tumor penetration within the colonic wall [2]. Although final stage classification is deferred to review of permanent sections, pathologists may be asked to provide intraoperative staging information in some cases, such as assessment of apparently superficial lesions, which may be amenable to local excision. Gross assessment of tumor invasion is best achieved by serially sectioning at close intervals, which usually allows one to estimate whether it is limited to the lamina propria, or penetrates the submucosa, muscularis propria, or serosa. Invasive carcinomas appear as tan-white, ill-defined masses that obliterate normal tissue layers of the colonic wall, and the deepest invasion usually occurs in the tumor epicenter [3] (Fig. 1.1).

The term "carcinoma in situ" is generally avoided as a diagnostic category in colorectal neoplasia because it encompasses both intraepithelial carcinoma and tumors that are invasive of the lamina propria but confined to the muscularis mucosae. Most pathologists prefer the term "adenoma with high-grade dysplasia" to describe a neoplastic proliferation confined to the basement membrane

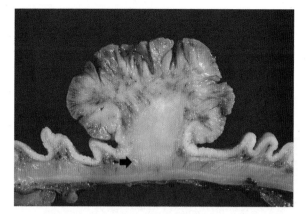

Fig. 1.1 Invasive adenocarcinoma within a polyp obliterates tissue planes between the mucosa and submucosa and superficially infiltrates the inner layer of the muscularis propria (*arrow*). The adjacent colonic wall shows a clear demarcation between the superficial mucosa, gelatinous submucosa, and both layers of the muscularis propria

(Fig. 1.2), and "intramucosal carcinoma" to describe tumors that do not extend beyond the muscularis mucosae [4] (Fig. 1.3).

Cancers that extend into the submucosa (pT1) are generally detected in polypectomy specimens, since these early, often asymptomatic, tumors are identified during screening or surveillance colonoscopy. One potential pitfall to the diagnosis of submucosal invasion is commonly observed in distally located adenomas that are subjected to luminal trauma (Fig. 1.4), or those that have been endoscopically manipulated in a prior procedure (Fig. 1.5). Traumatized adenomas may display epithelial misplacement into the polyp stalk, which has been termed "pseudoinvasion". The histologic distinction between invasive carcinoma and "pseudoinvasive" epithelium has significant clinical implications, since some patients with malignant polyps require a colectomy, whereas adenomas with epithelial misplacement are treated by polypectomy [5]. A variety of morphologic features help distinguish adenomas with misplaced epithelium from those with invasive adenocarcinoma. Misplaced epithelium resembles that present in the

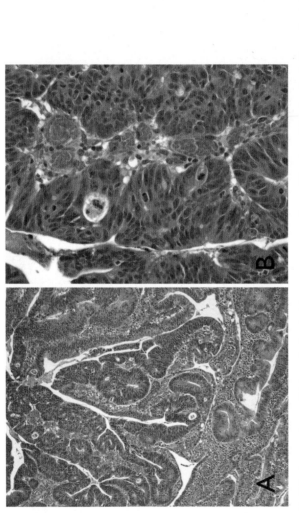

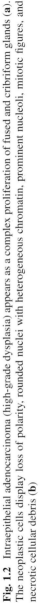

Fig. 1.2 Intraepithelial adenocarcinoma (high-grade dysplasia) appears as a complex proliferation of fused and cribriform glands (**a**). The neoplastic cells display loss of polarity, rounded nuclei with heterogeneous chromatin, prominent nucleoli, mitotic figures, and necrotic cellular debris (**b**)

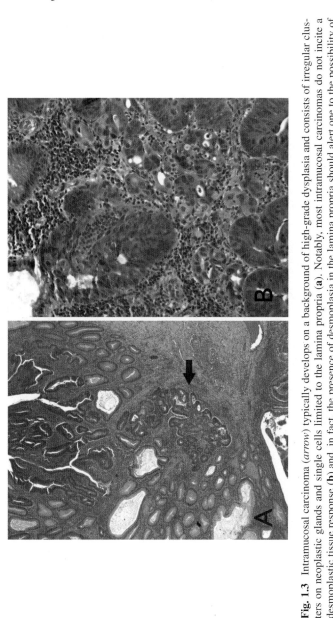
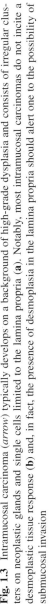

Fig. 1.3 Intramucosal carcinoma (*arrow*) typically develops on a background of high-grade dysplasia and consists of irregular clusters on neoplastic glands and single cells limited to the lamina propria (**a**). Notably, most intramucosal carcinomas do not incite a desmoplastic tissue response (**b**) and, in fact, the presence of desmoplasia in the lamina propria should alert one to the possibility of submucosal invasion

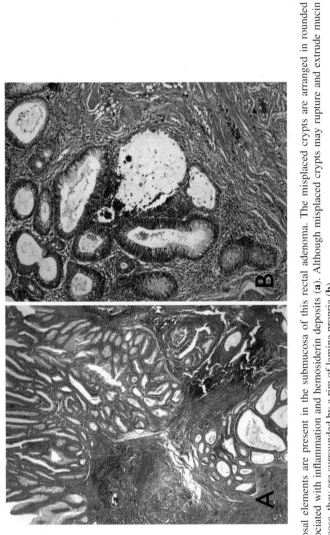

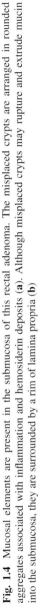

Fig. 1.4 Mucosal elements are present in the submucosa of this rectal adenoma. The misplaced crypts are arranged in rounded aggregates associated with inflammation and hemosiderin deposits (**a**). Although misplaced crypts may rupture and extrude mucin into the submucosa, they are surrounded by a rim of lamina propria (**b**)

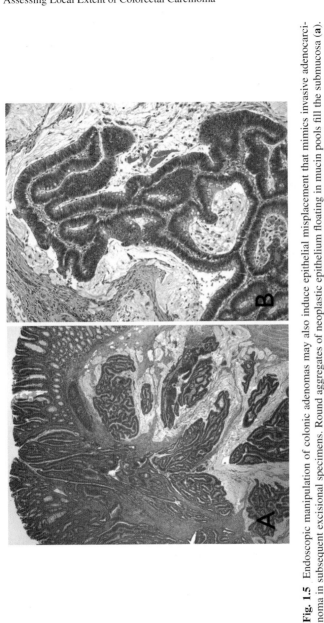
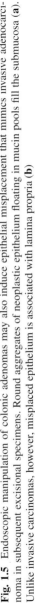

Fig. 1.5 Endoscopic manipulation of colonic adenomas may also induce epithelial misplacement that mimics invasive adenocarcinoma in subsequent excisional specimens. Round aggregates of neoplastic epithelium floating in mucin pools fill the submucosa (**a**). Unlike invasive carcinomas, however, misplaced epithelium is associated with lamina propria (**b**)

mucosal component and is accompanied by a distinct rim of lamina propria [6] (Fig. 1.4). The crypts dilate and rupture, inciting an inflammatory response to extruded mucin, and stromal hemorrhage with hemosiderin deposits is common. In contrast, adenocarcinomas grow in an infiltrative pattern, are not accompanied by lamina propria tissue, and incite a desmoplastic stromal response (Fig. 1.6a). Invasive epithelial cells are cytologically atypical with high-grade nuclei, nuclear pleomorphism, and clumped chromatin (Fig. 1.6b).

The distinction between carcinomas that invade, but are limited to, the muscularis propria (pT2) and those that extend into the pericolic or subserosal adipose tissue (pT3) is generally straightforward. The minimal criteria for pT3 classification include an absence of smooth muscle cells of the muscularis propria between the leading edge of the tumor and the pericolic fat [2].

The most problematic aspect of tumor stage assignment is the recognition of pT4 lesions. This stage is subdivided into two categories: pT4a is now defined as serosal penetration, whereas pT4b denotes direct tumor extension into another organ. Serosal penetration produces shaggy, fibrinous serosal adhesions, often with puckering, although some cases may show complete penetration and perforation of the serosal surface (Fig. 1.7a). Serosal involvement may be detected by scraping the serosa and smearing the material on a glass slide or touching a glass slide to the serosal surface and staining the slide with hematoxylin and eosin. Cytology preparations obtained from the serosal surface contain clusters of neoplastic epithelial cells and a background of reactive mesothelial hyperplasia and inflammation (Fig. 1.7b). Serosal penetration is most readily recognized in histologic sections when free tumor cells are present on the serosal surface, or when tumor cells are present at the serosal surface in combination with mesothelial cell hyperplasia or an inflammatory reaction (Fig. 1.8a). The presence of tumor cells within close proximity of a mesothelial inflammatory reaction also predicts decreased survival, despite the apparent lack of tumor cells on the serosa, and most likely represents a tissue response to serosal penetration [7] (Fig. 1.8b). Note that the serosa is not a surgical margin and serosal penetration by tumor does not constitute an incomplete resection.

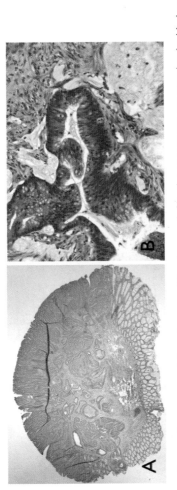

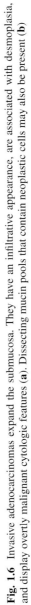

Fig. 1.6 Invasive adenocarcinomas expand the submucosa. They have an infiltrative appearance, are associated with desmoplasia, and display overtly malignant cytologic features (**a**). Dissecting mucin pools that contain neoplastic cells may also be present (**b**)

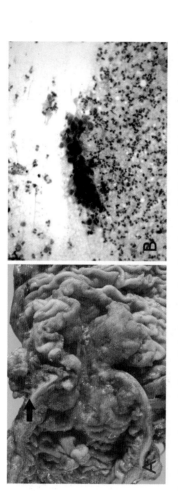

Fig. 1.7 Colonic adenocarcinomas that penetrate the serosal surface frequently display fibrinous adhesions on the serosa (*arrow*) directly subjacent to the tumor (**a**). Serosal penetration is easily documented by creating cytologic preparations from material obtained by touching, or scraping, the serosal surface of the fresh specimen. Neoplastic epithelial cells form cohesive groups on a background of inflammation (**b**)

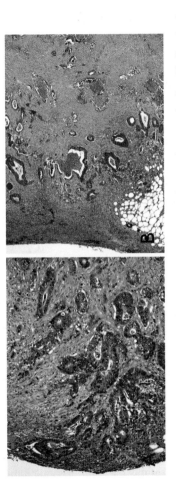

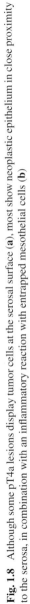

Fig. 1.8 Although some pT4a lesions display tumor cells at the serosal surface (**a**), most show neoplastic epithelium in close proximity to the serosa, in combination with an inflammatory reaction with entrapped mesothelial cells (**b**)

Assessing Lymph Node Status

Pathologists are rarely asked to assess lymph node status during colon cancer surgery, although one may occasionally receive non-regional lymph nodes for frozen section diagnosis. The regional lymph nodes for colorectal carcinomas are staged as pN0, pN1, or pN2 depending upon the number of lymph nodes involved by carcinoma. Notably, non-regional lymph nodes that contain tumor deposits should be staged as pM1 disease. There is no universal agreement regarding the minimum number of lymph nodes that should be retrieved in order to accurately predict the likelihood of regional node negativity, although removal and examination of at least twelve lymph nodes is generally considered adequate [8]. By convention, rounded tumor nodules within the pericolic fat that are discontinuous with the main tumor mass are considered to represent completely replaced lymph nodes even if no residual nodal tissue is identified.

Evaluation of Resection Margins

A number of problems arise when assessing surgical resection margins on colectomy specimens. Most issues are resolved following close examination of the specimen, review of the radiology report, and direct conversations with the surgeon. Common problems include inadvertent inclusion of the serosa as a resection margin and a failure to recognize the radial resection margin on rectal specimens. Every colonic resection specimen has at least three surgical resection margins:the proximal margin (which should be the ileum on proximal colonic resection specimens), the distal margin, and the radial margin. There is a very high correlation between the impression of margin status on gross examination and histologic findings. Extensive lateral, or submucosal, tumor spread is rare among primary colonic carcinomas, so gross examination of the proximal and distal margins is usually sufficient for margins distant (>3 cm) from the tumor [9]. Tumors present within 1 cm of the margin should be evaluated with perpendicular sections, whereas parallel (*en face*) sections may be obtained in cases that display greater tumor clearance. Close margins are commonly encountered among low-lying rectal cancers, since it may be difficult for the surgeon to obtain a wide margin while preserving anal sphincter function [10] (Fig. 1.9). Surgeons may also have a difficult time judging the status of the distal margin in the neoadjuvant setting, since the residual tumor may be small (Fig. 1.10).

The radial margin is a soft tissue resection margin reflecting either transection of the mesentery, or a surgical plane of dissection, and its nature varies depending on the anatomic location of the tumor and the type of surgical specimen obtained. The radial

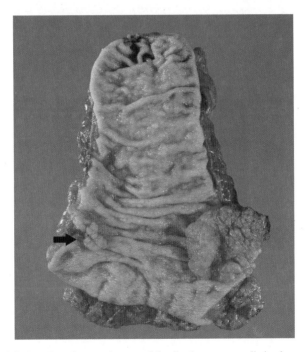

Fig. 1.9 Invasive adenocarcinomas of the distal rectum may lie in close proximity to the distal resection margin, and thus, surgeons commonly request gross examination of the specimen by pathologists in order to assure adequate tumor clearance. Note the additional presence of a smaller polyp in this resection specimen (*arrow*)

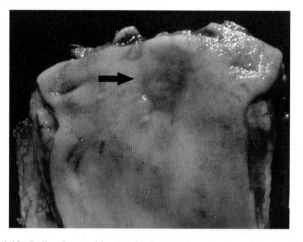

Fig. 1.10 Bulky, inoperable rectal adenocarcinomas may show a striking response to neoadjuvant therapy, such that the residual lesion appears as an ulcer associated with mural scarring (*arrow*). Tumors that occur in the most distal rectum may be excised with a narrow margin in order to preserve the anal sphincter. Intraoperative evaluation of close margins should include parallel sections of the tumor in relation to the distal margin

margin of colonic segments that lie within the peritoneal cavity (cecum, transverse colon, and sigmoid colon) is the mesenteric resection margin. Segments of colon located partially within the peritoneal cavity (ascending colon and descending colon) are surfaced anteriorly by peritoneum but lie on the posterior abdominal wall. Therefore, the radial margins of cancers that occur in these areas include both the mesenteric margin and the posterior aspect of the specimen [2].

In contrast, the radial resection margin of the rectum is a circumferential margin because it lies below the peritoneal reflection. The results of several studies have shown that the status of this margin is a powerful predictor of local recurrence and is probably the most important margin on rectal cancer resection specimens [11]. The adipose tissue surrounding the lower two-thirds of the rectum is enveloped by delicate fibroconnective tissue, termed the mesorectum, which may be sharply dissected from adjacent pelvic structures. The mesorectum begins below the peritoneal reflection in the upper rectum where it is limited to the posterior aspect of the rectum and is continuous with the sigmoid mesocolon [12] (Fig. 1.11). Advances in surgical techniques over the past few decades have led to the widespread practice of total mesorectal excision for rectal carcinoma. In this situation, the surgeon dissects the rectum along the areolar plane outside the mesorectal fascia, such that the rectum, mesorectum, and all regional lymph nodes are removed entirely [13]. This surgical technique decreases the risk of local recurrence and improves overall survival, so pathologists may be called upon to comment on the intactness of the mesorectal envelope in cancer cases [11, 14, 15] (Fig. 1.12). Evaluation

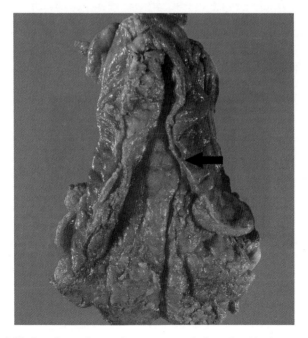

Fig. 1.11 Rectal resection specimens are posteriorly surfaced by the mesorectum, which represents a surgical margin. The mesorectum lies inferior to the peritoneal reflection (*arrow*) and tapers proximally but is broader in the lower two-thirds of the specimen

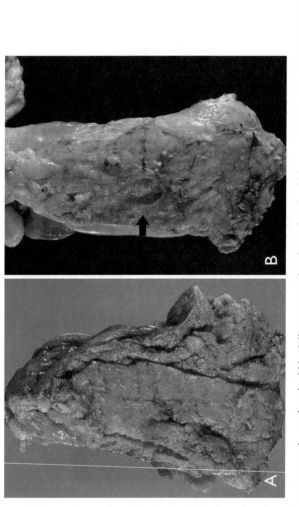
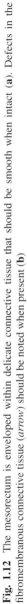

Fig. 1.12 The mesorectum is enveloped within delicate connective tissue that should be smooth when intact (**a**). Defects in the fibromembranous connective tissue (*arrow*) should be noted when present (**b**)

of the mesorectum should always be performed on an unopened specimen in the fresh state. Assessment should include evaluation of smoothness of the mesorectal surface, tissue bulk, and documentation of the presence of defects in the mesorectal fascia [16] (Table 1.1).

Table 1.1 Pathologic classification of mesorectal excision adequacy

Complete	■ Mesorectum intact and smooth
	■ If present, defects span <5 mm
Nearly complete	■ Slightly irregular mesorectal fascia
	■ Defects in mesorectal fat do not extend into muscularis propria
Incomplete	■ Small amount of mesorectal connective tissue
	■ Defects in mesorectal fat extend into muscularis propria
	■ Coning of distal soft tissue
	■ Irregular radial margin on sectioning

Implications of Neoadjuvant Therapy

Surgeons may request intraoperative consultations on resection specimens from patients who have undergone preoperative radiation and/or chemoradiation, in order to determine the status of the mesorectal and distal margins. Neoadjuvantly treated rectal cancers may appear as a mucosal pucker or shallow ulcer overlying mural fibrosis (Fig. 1.13). In this situation, careful documentation of the status of the radial (Fig. 1.14) and distal margins (Fig. 1.15) with frozen sections is warranted, since residual carcinoma at the margin may be difficult to distinguish from posttreatment scarring by gross inspection alone [10]. Importantly, acellular mucin pools in neoadjuvantly treated patients are considered to represent complete tumor response and are not used to assign pathologic stage (Fig. 1.16).

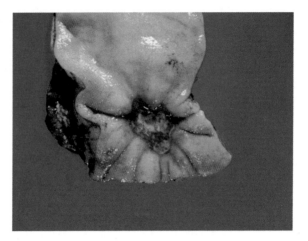

Fig. 1.13 A mucosal ulcer near the distal resection margin remains following neoadjuvant therapy. In this situation, perpendicular sections that demonstrate the relationship between the distal margin and residual tumor should be obtained to document adequate resection. The entire ulcer and subjacent colonic wall should be submitted for histologic evaluation, since tumor regression following therapy is an important predictor of outcome

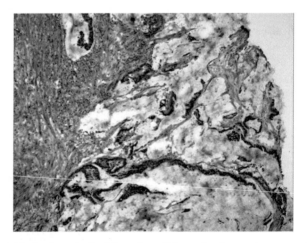

Fig. 1.14 Sections obtained from the radial margin of a rectal cancer patient display infiltrative adenocarcinoma associated with mucin pools, enmeshed within fibroinflammatory stroma

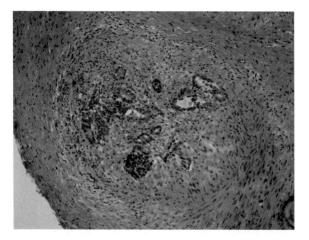

Fig. 1.15 Neoadjuvantly treated cancers of the distal rectum are often excised with a narrow margin that may be evaluated with frozen section, when appropriate. In this case, an ulcer was present 1 cm from the distal margin, but frozen section demonstrated microscopic foci of residual cancer at the resection margin

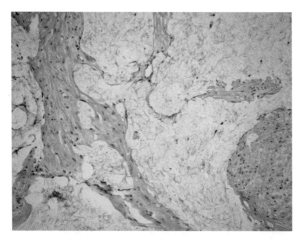

Fig. 1.16 Tumor regression is often manifest as acellular mucin pools within the rectal wall. Although their presence reflects the pre-treatment extent of the cancer, acellular mucin pools should not be used to assign pathologic stage to neoadjuvantly treated rectal cancers

References

1. Jemal A, Siegal R, Ward E, et al (2008) Cancer statistics. CA Cancer J Clin 58(2):71–96
2. Washington MK, Berlin J, Branton P, et al (2009) Protocol for the examination of specimens from patients with primary carcinomas of the colon and rectum. Arch Pathol Lab Med 133:1539–1551
3. Burroughs SH, Williams GT (2000) Examination of large intestine resection specimens. J Clin Pathol 53:344–349
4. Terry MB, Neugut AI, Bostick RM, Potter JD, Haile RW, Fenoglio-Preiser CM (2002) Reliability in the classification of advanced colorectal adenomas. Cancer Epidemiol Biomarkers Prev 11(7):660–663
5. Ramirez M, Scherling S, Papaconstantinou HT, Scott TJ (2008) Management of the malignant polyp. Clin Colon Rectal Surg 21(4): 286–290
6. Yantiss RK, Bosenberg MW, Antonioli DA, and Odze RD (2002) Utility of MMP-1, p53, E-cadherin, and collagen IV immunohistochemical stains in the differential diagnosis of adenomas with misplaced epithelium versus adenomas with invasive adenocarcinoma. Am J Surg Pathol 26(2):206–215
7. Shepherd NA, Baxter KJ, Love SB (1997) The prognostic importance of peritoneal involvement in colonic cancer: a prospective evaluation. Gastroenterology 112(4):1096–1102
8. Scott KW, Grace RH (1989) Detection of lymph node metastases in colorectal carcinoma before and after fat clearance. Br J Surg 76(11): 1165–1167
9. Hughes TG, Jenevein EP, Poulos E (1983) Intramural spread of colon carcinoma. A pathologic study. Am J Surg 46(3):697–699
10. Luna-Perez P, Huelga AR, Coria DFR, Medrano R, Macouzet JG (1990) Usefulness of frozen section examination in resected mid-rectal cancer after preoperative radiation. Am J Surg 159(6):582–584
11. Kapiteijn E, Marijnen CA, Nagtegaal ID, et al (2005) Preoperative radiotherapy combined with total mesorectal excision for resectable rectal cancer. N Engl J Med 345(9):638–646
12. Salerno G, Daniels IR, Moran BJ, Wotherspoon A, Brown G (2006) Clarifying margins in the multidisciplinary management of rectal cancer: the MERCURY experience. Clin Radiol 61(11):916–923
13. Wasserberg N, Gutman H (2008) Resection margins in modern rectal cancer surgery. J Surg Oncol 98(8):611–615
14. Arbman G, Nilsson E, Hallböök O, Sjödahl R (1996) Local recurrence following total mesorectal excision for rectal cancer. Eur J Surg 162(11):899–904
15. Nagtegaal ID, vandeVeld CJ, vanderWorp E, Kapiteijn E, Quirke P, van Krieken JH (2002) Macroscopic evaluation of rectal cancer resection specimens: clinical significance of the pathologist in quality control. J Clin Oncol 20(7):1729–1734
16. Hermanek P, Junginger T (2005) The circumferential resection margin in rectal carcinoma. Tech Coloproctol 9(3):193–200

Chapter 2
Intraoperative Evaluation for Extracolonic Disease in Colon Cancer Patients

Abstract Although radiographic studies usually provide accurate preoperative staging information in colorectal cancer patients, intraoperative frozen section evaluation of extracolonic tissues may be requested in order to confirm the diagnosis of a metastasis or ensure its complete resection. The liver represents the most common site of distant organ metastases from colorectal cancer. Several benign lesions may simulate liver metastases, most notably von Meyenberg complexes and bile duct hamartomas. Peritoneal carcinomatosis is also an important intraoperative finding that may alter the surgical management of colon cancer patients. A number of mimics of peritoneal carcinomatosis are encountered in the frozen section laboratory.

Keywords Metastasis · Liver · Bile duct hamartoma · Peritoneal carcinomatosis

Introduction

Radiographic studies provide accurate preoperative staging information for most colorectal cancer patients, although surgeons may observe unsuspected abnormalities during exploratory laparotomy that warrant intraoperative consultation. Frozen section evaluation of extracolonic tissues may be requested by the surgeon in order to

N.C. Panarelli, R.K. Yantiss, *Frozen Section Library: Appendix,*   21
Colon, and Anus, Frozen Section Library 4, DOI 10.1007/978-1-4419-6584-4_2,
© Springer Science+Business Media, LLC 2010

confirm a diagnosis of metastasis, ensure complete resection of a metastatic deposit, or to make a diagnosis on a newly discovered lesion. Thus, it is important for pathologists to be familiar with the morphologic characteristics of colorectal carcinoma, as well as those of a variety of entities that may simulate the appearance of a metastasis.

Liver Metastases

Gross Features

The liver is the most common site of distant organ metastasis from colorectal cancer, and up to 25% of patients with colon cancer have liver metastases at the time of surgery. However, unlike many cancer patients, some individuals with colorectal carcinoma may undergo resection of limited liver metastases, since this procedure improves outcome in a subset of patients. The aim of surgery is complete tumor resection with maximal preservation of liver function [1]. Therefore, intraoperative evaluation may be required to determine the adequacy of hepatic resection [2]. Hepatic metastases of colorectal carcinoma typically appear as one, or more, relatively well-circumscribed tan, white nodules unassociated with cirrhosis (Fig. 2.1). They may have a depressed, variegated cut surface owing to the presence of extensive necrosis.

Microscopic Features

Colorectal cancer metastases usually consist of overtly malignant infiltrative glands, many of which contain abundant necrotic luminal debris (Fig. 2.2). Most show a variable amount of desmoplastic stroma surrounding tumor cells, although the stroma may show hyalinization, particularly when patients have received prior chemotherapy. Tumors that have been treated with embolization may be entirely non-viable.

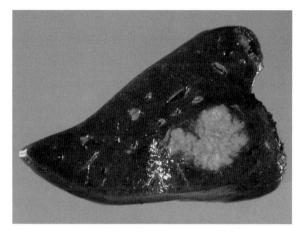

Fig. 2.1 Metastatic colorectal cancer deposits are *pale yellow*, or *white*, with a loculated rim. They may contain depressions that reflect tumor necrosis. The amount of resected liver is largely determined by the anatomic location of metastases, although margins may be close in order to maximally preserve hepatic function

Differential Diagnosis

Several benign liver lesions may simulate colorectal cancer metastases [3–8] (Table 2.1). Most are detected during laparotomy and, thus, may prompt intraoperative consultation. The most common entities to consider in the differential diagnosis of metastatic carcinoma include von Meyenberg complexes (bile duct hamartomas) and biliary adenomas [2]. Both types of lesions appear as small, tan-white nodules, which may be multiple (Fig. 2.3). Bile duct hamartomas are well-circumscribed proliferations of variably cystic ductules enmeshed within hyalized stroma. The ducts are lined by flattened, or cuboidal, epithelium without cytologic atypia and may contain bile plugs (Fig. 2.4). Biliary adenomas contain a proliferation of small bile ductules within compact, cellular stroma. The ductules are lined by bland cuboidal epithelial cells with mild cytologic atypia and generally do not contain bile (Fig. 2.5).

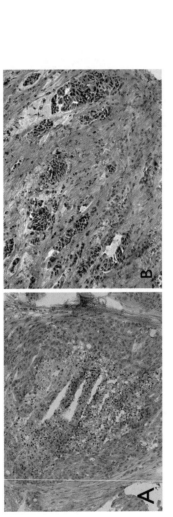

Fig. 2.2 Metastatic colorectal cancer deposits are composed of malignant glands that contain abundant luminal necrotic debris (**a**) or are enmeshed within desmoplastic stroma (**b**)

Table 2.1 Mimics of metastatic colorectal carcinoma in the liver

- Von Meyenberg complex
    - Often multiple
    - Firm, white subcapsular nodules
    - Cystic ducts lined by bland, flattened epithelium
    - Dense, hyalinized stroma
    - Bile often present in ductules
    - No atypia, mitoses, or necrosis
- Biliary adenoma
    - Often multiple
    - Well-circumscribed, firm, grey-white subcapsular nodules with central depression
    - Compact proliferation of small tubular ducts with a abundant cytoplasm and pale nuclei
    - Lack cystic dilatation and bile
    - No atypia, mitoses, or necrosis
- Hemangioma
- Multifocal fatty infiltration
    - Multiple radiographically apparent spherical densities
    - Macrovesicular steatosis in liver biopsy material
- Solitary necrotic nodule of the liver
    - Necrotic core surrounded by hyalinized fibrotic tissue
- Abscess
- Extrinsic compression by primary neoplasm or diaphragmatic implants

Peritoneal Disease

Peritoneal carcinomatosis describes widespread intra-abdominal metastases and, with the exception of low-grade appendiceal mucinous neoplasms, is not amenable to surgical debulking. In fact, detection of peritoneal metastases during exploratory laparotomy impacts the subsequent management of the patient and may alter the surgical procedure, so intraoperative evaluation plays a vital role in the care of patients with suspected tumor involvement of the peritoneal cavity [1, 9, 10]. Peritoneal carcinomatosis may appear as gray, or white, nodules within the peritoneal fat or studding the serosal surfaces of the viscera (Fig. 2.6). Colorectal cancers with mucinous differentiation disseminate in the form of implants comprised of pools of mucin that contain neoplastic

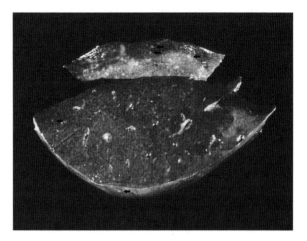

Fig. 2.3 Von Meyenberg complexes are round, *gray-white* nodules that may be multiple (*arrows*). Most are subcapsular and, thus, evident to the surgeon, who may submit them for frozen section analysis

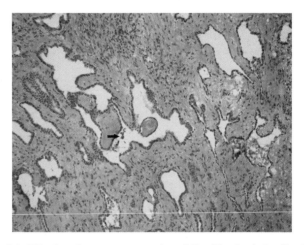

Fig. 2.4 Bile duct hamartomas contain mildly dilated tubules lined by cuboidal, or attenuated, epithelial cells without atypia. Occasional tubules may contain bile (*arrow*). The surrounding stroma is eosinophilic and rich in collagen, which may be hyalinized

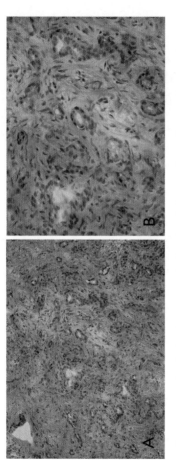

Fig. 2.5 Bile duct adenomas may closely simulate metastatic deposits of adenocarcinoma because they contain numerous proliferating tubules enmeshed within cellular stroma (**a**). However, the lesional cells are cytologically bland and contain abundant cytoplasm with uniform, pale nuclei (**b**)

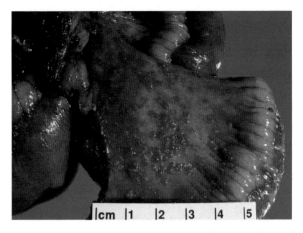

Fig. 2.6 *Pale pink* or *gray* nodules on the visceral serosa reflect peritoneal carcinomatosis. Cancers with striking desmoplasia are firm and gritty, whereas those with mucin production are soft and gelatinous

epithelial cells arranged singly or in nests and glands (Fig. 2.7). Tumor cells typically show marked cytologic atypia and mitotic activity, although mucinous neoplasms derived from the appendix may appear deceptively bland, resulting in considerable diagnostic confusion, as discussed in Chapter 6.

Differential Diagnosis

Two common mimics of peritoneal carcinomatosis may be encountered in samples submitted for frozen section analysis because both may grossly appear as one or more ill-defined gray, or white, nodules within peritoneal fat or on the intestinal serosa (Fig. 2.8). Mesenteric fat necrosis may simulate the appearance of metastatic poorly differentiated carcinoma, since the aggregates of macrophages display abundant cytoplasm and may show patchy cytologic atypia (Fig. 2.9a). Clues to the diagnosis include the presence of fat vacuoles surrounded by macrophages, mixed inflammation, dystrophic calcifications, and multinucleated cells

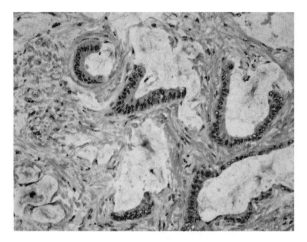

Fig. 2.7 Peritoneal deposits of mucinous carcinoma consist of dissecting mucin pools, some of which contain strips or clusters of malignant epithelium. Overtly malignant tumor deposits such as this one are not amenable to surgical debulking or peritoneal stripping

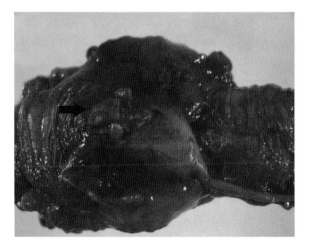

Fig. 2.8 Fat necrosis may appear as *yellow-white* lobulated excrescences on the serosal surface (*arrow*)

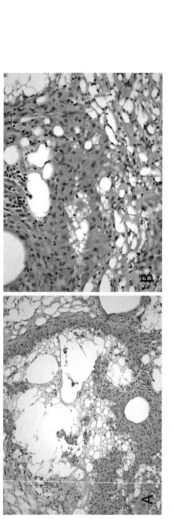

Fig. 2.9 Sheets of macrophages in fat necrosis may simulate the appearance of carcinoma (**a**). Clues to the diagnosis include the presence of mixed background inflammation and variably sized vesicles of extracellular fat (**b**)

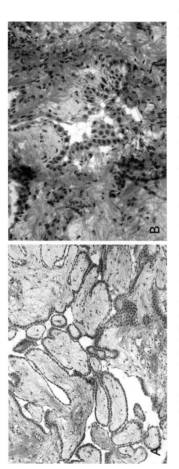

Fig. 2.10 Papillary mesothelial hyperplasia is limited to the peritoneal surfaces and consists of an exuberant proliferation of mesothelial cells. Papillae contain loose fibrous connective tissue and are lined by a single layer of mesothelium (**a**). Mesothelial cells contain abundant eosinophilic cytoplasm and small, round nuclei without appreciable mitotic activity (**b**)

(Fig. 2.9b). Benign mesothelial proliferations, such as localized papillary mesothelial hyperplasia and reactive mesothelial hyperplasia, contain mildly atypical mesothelial cells that display complex architectural growth patterns (Fig. 2.10a). These lesions should be readily distinguished from metastatic colonic carcinomas, since the latter generally metastasize in the form of infiltrating glands and single cells. Most colorectal carcinomas also show overtly malignant cytologic features with nuclear irregularities and hyperchromasia, whereas mesothelial cells have abundant eosinophilic cytoplasm and uniform, round nuclei evident upon frozen section analysis (Fig. 2.10b). Epithelial cell proliferations of Mullerian derivation may simulate the appearance of peritoneal carcinomatosis and are discussed more fully in Chapter 3. Common benign mimics of metastatic carcinoma to the peritoneal cavity are enumerated in Table 2.2 [11–13].

Table 2.2 Peritoneal lesions that may simulate peritoneal carcinomatosis

- Mesenteric and omental fat necrosis
- Mesothelial lesions
  - Cysts
  - Localized papillary hyperplasia
  - Mesothelial hyperplasia with reactive atypia
- Peritoneal infections (*Mycobacterium tuberculosis*, *Actinomyces*)
- Endometriosis
- Florid endosalpingiosis

References

1. Cao CQ, Yan TD, Liauw W, Morris DL (2009) Comparison of optimally resected hepatectomy and peritonectomy patient with colorectal cancer metastasis. J Surg Oncol 100(7):529–533
2. Rakha E, Ramaiah S, McGregor A (2006) Accuracy of frozen section in the diagnosis of liver mass lesions. J Clin Pathol 59:352–354
3. Citak EC, Karadeniz C, Oguz A, Boyunaga O, Ekinci O, Okur V (2007) Nodular regenerative hyperplasia and focal nodular hyperplasia of the liver mimicking hepatic metastasis in children with solid tumors and a review of literature. Pediatr Hematol Oncol 24(4):281–289

4. Kondi-Pafiti AI, Grapsa DS, Kairi-Vasilatou ED, Voros DK, Smyrniotis VE (2006) "Solitary necrotic nodule of the liver": an enigmatic entity mimicking malignancy. Int J Gastrointest Cancer 37(23):74–78

5. Kroncke TJ, Taupitz M, Kivelitz D, et al (2000) Multifocal nodular fatty infiltration of the liver mimicking metastatic disease on CT: imaging findings and diagnosis using MR imaging. Eur Radiol 10(7):1095–1100

6. Ryan RS, Al-Hashimi H, Lee MJ (2001) Hepatic abscesses in elderly patients mimicking metastatic disease. Ir J Med Sci 170(4):251–253

7. Yamashita Y, Shimada M, Taguchi K, et al (2000) Hepatic sclerosing hemangioma mimicking a metastatic liver tumor: report of a case. Surg Today 30(9):849–852

8. Yoon KH, Yun KJ, Lee JM, Kim CG (2000) Solitary necrotic nodules of the liver mimicking hepatic metastases: report of two cases. Korean J Radiol 1(3):165–168

9. Varban O, Levine EA, Stewart JH, McCoy TP, Shen P (2009) Outcomes associated with cytoreductive surgery and intraperitoneal hyperthermic chemotherapy in colorectal patients with peritoneal surface disease and hepatic metastases. Cancer 115(15):3427–3436

10. DeHaas RJ, Wicherts DA, Adam R (2008) Resection of colorectal liver metastases with extrahepatic disease. Dig Surg 25(6):461–466

11. Clement PB, Granai CO, Young RH, Scully RE (1994) Endometriosis with myxoid change. A case simulating pseudomyxoma peritonei. Am J Surg Pathol 18(8):849–853

12. Hameed A, Jafri N, Copeland LJ, O'Toole RV (1996) Endometriosis with myxoid change simulating mucinous adenocarcinoma and pseudomyxoma peritonei. Gynecol Oncol 62(2):317–319

13. Ozan H, Ozerkan K, Orhan A (2009) Peritoneal tuberculosis mimicking peritoneal carcinomatosis. Eur J Gynaecol Oncol 30(4):426–430

Chapter 3
Metastases and Mimics of Colorectal Carcinoma

Abstract Secondary involvement of the colon by other malignant neoplasms may mimic primary colorectal carcinoma and results from direct extension, peritoneal seeding, or hematogenous spread. Careful gross examination and key histologic features may suggest the presence of a metastasis. Most primary tumors are solitary mucosa-based lesions, whereas secondary neoplasms may be multiple and often substantially affect the outer colonic wall. Primary colorectal cancers are comprised of malignant cribriform glands with necrosis and show dysplasia in the overlying mucosa, whereas secondary tumors show variable growth patterns and readily detectable lymphovascular invasion. Several benign processes, namely diverticulitis and intestinal endometriosis, may also mimic colon cancers and their nature may not be apparent prior to surgical intervention.

Keywords Metastasis · Diverticulitis · Endometriosis · Mimics · Colorectal · Carcinoma

Introduction

A number of malignant neoplasms may secondarily involve the colon via direct extension, peritoneal seeding, or hematogenous spread, thereby simulating the appearance of a primary carcinoma.

N.C. Panarelli, R.K. Yantiss, *Frozen Section Library: Appendix,*
Colon, and Anus, Frozen Section Library 4, DOI 10.1007/978-1-4419-6584-4_3,
© Springer Science+Business Media, LLC 2010

The most common sources of metastases to the colon among women include primary tumors of the gynecologic tract, breast, and lung, whereas metastases from the extracolonic gastrointestinal tract and lung are most common among men. The colon may also be a site of metastasis, or direct extension, for carcinomas of the bladder, kidneys, pancreas, prostate, and cervix, and malignant melanoma of the skin or anus. Women may develop Mullerian malignancies derived from endometriotic foci within the colon or, more frequently, colonic endometriosis may simulate the appearance of colonic carcinoma.

The possibility of an extracolonic malignancy is generally suspected at the time of surgery, owing to the widespread use of imaging techniques and endoscopically obtained mucosal biopsies prior to the surgical procedure. However, intraoperative frozen section analysis may be requested in order to distinguish primary colorectal carcinoma from metastases, since the latter may not be resected. Colonic involvement by an extra-intestinal malignancy may, rarely, represent the initial presentation of a tumor of unknown origin, particularly when dealing with carcinomas of the breast and metastatic melanoma. Although it is often impossible to determine the site of origin based on frozen section analysis alone, the pathologist may provide information that will guide the clinical management of the patient. Finally, hematopoetic malignancies may simulate the gross and endoscopic appearance of colonic carcinomas. These tumors require appropriate triaging of materials for flow cytometry and subsequent molecular studies, as discussed in Chapter 4.

Primary Colorectal Cancer Versus Secondary Malignancies of the Colon

Gross Features of Colorectal Carcinoma

Most colorectal adenocarcinomas are solitary exophytic, polypoid tumors, or endophytic, ulcerative lesions based in the mucosa and submucosa (Fig. 3.1). Serosal involvement is generally limited,

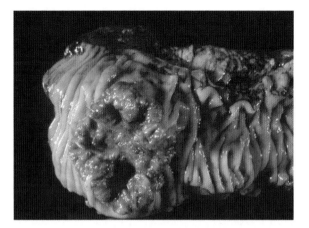

Fig. 3.1 Primary colonic adenocarcinomas are usually polypoid or plaquelike mucosa-based tumors with a central depression or ulcer

and, in fact, one should be suspicious of a secondary neoplasm if its epicenter lies in the outer aspect of the colonic wall. Some colorectal carcinomas may be multifocal, particularly among patients with underlying polyposis disorders, but one should be suspicious of a metastasis if more than two tumor nodules are present. Notably, multiple adenomas, or underlying inflammatory bowel disease, are suggestive of primary colorectal carcinoma (Fig. 3.2).

Microscopic Features of Colorectal Carcinoma

Infiltrative cancers may be associated with apparent dysplasia overlying the tumor, however, one should be cautious when regarding this finding as a "hard" criterion for a primary malignancy, since colonization of the basement membrane may simulate the appearance of an in situ lesion, as described below (Fig. 3.3). Most colorectal adenocarcinomas consist of infiltrating single, or cribriform, glands with luminal necrosis and lack architectural heterogeneity (Fig. 3.4). Lymphovascular invasion is usually difficult

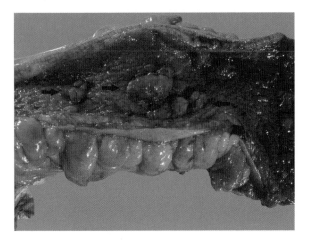

Fig. 3.2 Some colonic adenocarcinomas develop in patients with underlying inflammatory bowel disease and may be multifocal (*arrows*). The colitic mucosa displays mucosal nodularity, atrophy, and pseudopolyps, all of which should be extensively sampled to detect foci of dysplasia and/or early cancers

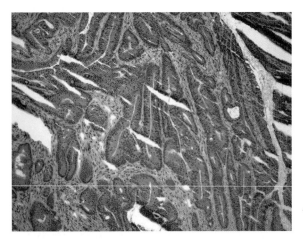

Fig. 3.3 The mucosa overlying invasive colorectal carcinomas typically contains neoplastic epithelium with basally located, pseudostratified nuclei with hyperchromasia and increased mitotic activity typical of an adenoma

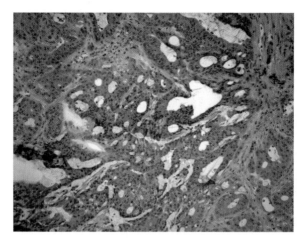

Fig. 3.4 Colorectal carcinomas contain a relatively homogeneous population of malignant glands, some of which show cystic dilation or cribriform architecture. The cells harbor abundant eosinophilic cytoplasm and round nuclei with coarse chromatin and prominent nucleoli. Mitotic figures and necrotic epithelial cells are easily identified

to detect, so its presence in abundance should raise suspicion for a metastasis.

Gross Features Suggestive of a Secondary Neoplasm

Tumors that directly invade the colon, or spread hematogenously, tend to involve the outer layers of the bowel wall with relative sparing of the mucosa (Fig. 3.5). Transmural tumor deposits may ulcerate and simulate a primary carcinoma, but they are ill-defined and undermine the mucosa upon careful inspection [1, 2] (Fig. 3.6). Malignant melanoma typically shows extensive lymphovascular invasion and fills the mucosa and submucosa, thereby producing a polypoid mass [3] (Fig. 3.7). Both mammary carcinoma and malignant melanoma may metastasize in the form of multiple nodules. Carcinomas of the gynecologic and extracolonic gastrointestinal tract are often associated with peritoneal disease.

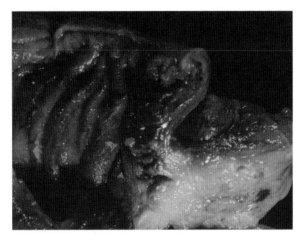

Fig. 3.5 Metastatic serous carcinoma extensively involves the pericolic fat and laterally invades the colonic wall. Although the lumen is nearly obstructed, minimal mucosal disease is present

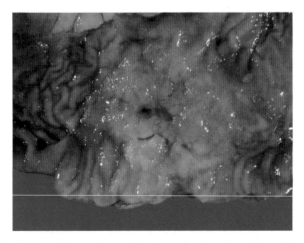

Fig. 3.6 Metastatic mammary carcinoma undermines the mucosa, distorting the normal folds. The ulcerated tumor has an irregular appearance

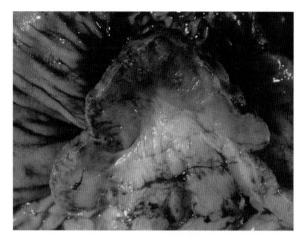

Fig. 3.7 Metastatic malignant melanoma extensively involves the mucosa and submucosa, producing a polypoid mass. Although pigmentation may be a helpful clue to the diagnosis, as in this case, up to half of gastrointestinal metastases are amelanotic

Microscopic Features Suggestive of a Secondary Neoplasm

Secondary malignancies of the colon commonly involve the serosal surface and outer muscularis propria to a greater degree than the inner bowel wall, and may show striking lymphovascular invasion (Fig. 3.8). Gland-forming tumors that invade the basement membrane from below may appear to mature, thereby simulating the appearance of an adenoma (Fig. 3.9). However, careful inspection reveals high-grade nuclear features not typically observed in most colorectal adenomas (Fig. 3.10). Mixed architectural growth patterns, including papillae, acini, and solid nests are quite unusual in colonic carcinomas, so a combination of these features should raise concern for an extra-intestinal neoplasm (Fig. 3.11). Colorectal carcinomas also show relatively high-grade nuclear features, despite extensive glandular differentiation, whereas other types of gland-forming tumors tend to contain less atypical nuclei (Fig. 3.12). Diffuse-type gastric cancers and

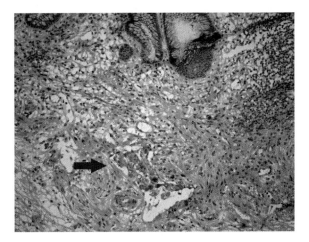

Fig. 3.8 Metastatic serous carcinoma extensively involves submucosal vascular spaces (*arrow*) and displays a greater degree of cytologic atypia than is usually observed in primary colorectal carcinomas

lobular breast cancers lack gland formation, but show low-grade nuclear features (Fig. 3.13), whereas metastatic melanomas display nucleolar prominence with abundant eosinophilic cytoplasm with, or without, pigmentation [1–3] (Fig. 3.14).

Some specific features are not typical of colorectal carcinoma, and their presence in frozen section slides should lead one to suspect a metastasis. Glands with slit-like spaces lined by cells with high-grade nuclei and prominent nucleoli should raise suspicion for serous carcinoma, especially if psammomatous calcifications are present (Fig. 3.15). Small glands with bland cytology and prominent nucleoli are characteristic of prostatic carcinomas. Solid tumors comprised of nests of tumor cells with a prominent vascular pattern may represent metastatic renal cell carcinoma or hepatocellular carcinoma. Although metastatic endometrioid carcinomas may be histologically indistinguishable from colonic carcinomas, those that arise from endometriosis generally display low-grade cytologic atypia and a background of endometriosis and atypical hyperplasia [4] (Fig. 3.16). Primary colonic squamous cell and adenosquamous carcinomas are extremely rare, so squamous

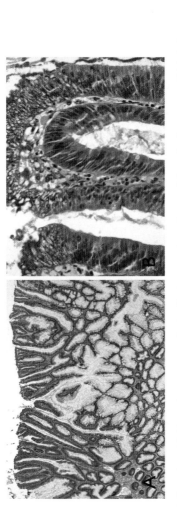

Fig. 3.9 Metastatic endometrioid carcinoma may colonize the basement membrane of the colonic mucosa, which induces apparent maturation of the neoplastic epithelium (**a**). The tumor cells contain abundant eosinophilic cytoplasm and cigar-shaped hyperchromatic nuclei similar to those observed in colonic adenomas (**b**)

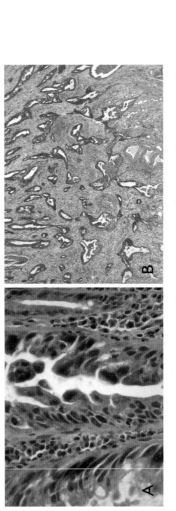

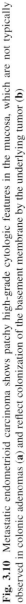

Fig. 3.10 Metastatic endometrioid carcinoma shows patchy high-grade cytologic features in the mucosa, which are not typically observed in colonic adenomas (**a**) and reflect colonization of the basement membrane by the underlying tumor (**b**)

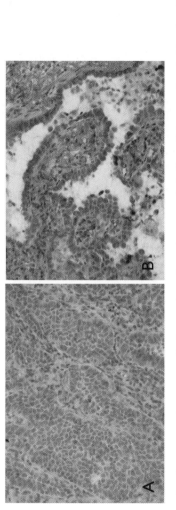
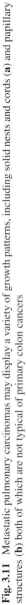

Fig. 3.11 Metastatic pulmonary carcinomas may display a variety of growth patterns, including solid nests and cords (**a**) and papillary structures (**b**) both of which are not typical of primary colon cancers

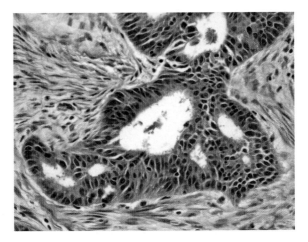

Fig. 3.12 Metastatic endometrioid carcinoma (same case as Figs. 3.8 and 3.9) contains cribriform glands, similar to colorectal carcinomas, but less cytologic atypia, and minimal, if any, mucin production

differentiation within an adenocarcinoma should alert one to the possibility of endometrioid carcinoma, particularly among female patients (Fig. 3.17). Distinguishing pathologic features of colorectal carcinoma and its neoplastic mimics are enumerated in Table 3.1.

Non-neoplastic Processes That Mimic Malignancy

Non-neoplastic processes induce a variety of mucosal and mural changes that simulate a mass lesion. Preoperative imaging studies may demonstrate findings concerning for a malignancy, yet mucosal biopsy samples obtained at colonoscopy often fail to yield a diagnosis. In this situation, surgeons might request intraoperative evaluation of biopsy samples, or the resection specimen, to guide further management.

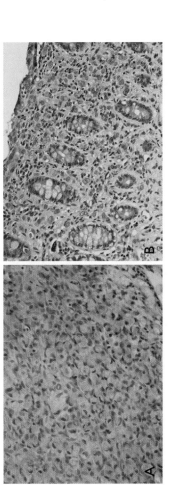
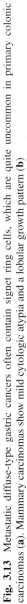

Fig. 3.13 Metastatic diffuse-type gastric cancers often contain signet ring cells, which are quite uncommon in primary colonic carcinomas (**a**). Mammary carcinomas show mild cytologic atypia and a lobular growth pattern (**b**)

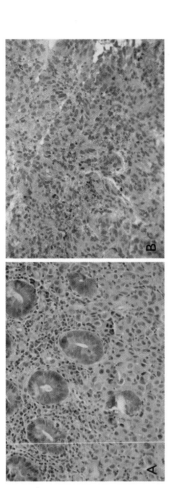

Fig. 3.14 Metastatic melanoma typically invades the colonic mucosa and infiltrate between colonic crypts. Melanoma cells contain abundant cytoplasm and large nuclei with prominent nucleoli (**a**). In contrast, diffuse-type colorectal carcinomas show high-grade cytologic features and harbor foci of cellular necrosis (**b**)

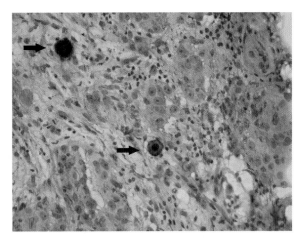

Fig. 3.15 Metastatic serous carcinoma in the colonic wall is associated with psammomatous calcifications (*arrows*). The tumor cells contain abundant eosinophilic cytoplasm and prominent nucleoli

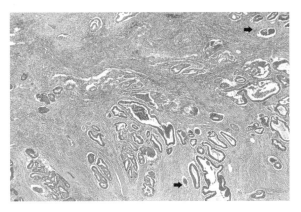

Fig. 3.16 Endometrioid adenocarcinomas derived from pre-existing colonic endometriosis are predominantly located within the colonic wall. These tumors arise on a background of benign endometriosis (*arrow*) and hyperplasia

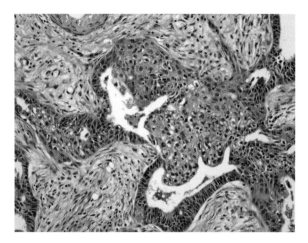

Fig. 3.17 Endometrioid adenocarcinomas frequently show squamous differentiation and, thus, the presence of this finding should prompt consideration of a secondary neoplasm in colonic resection specimens obtained from female patients

Diverticular Disease Associated Colitis

Patients with diverticulosis coli are at risk for complications, such as episodic diverticulitis, perforation, obstruction, and bleeding. Repetitive episodes of diverticulitis result in marked mural thickening, owing to a proliferation of smooth muscle cells in the muscularis propria, as well as post-inflammatory fibrosis which, in some cases, produces an indurated mass. Some cases are associated with striking mucosal redundancy and polyposis that simulates the appearance of a malignancy (Fig. 3.18a). Cross sectional sampling through these areas will demonstrate the presence of diverticula in combination with hypertrophy of the muscularis propria (Fig. 3.18b). The background mucosa may also show erythema and erosions and even display chronic colitis with fissuring ulcers and granulomas that mimic inflammatory bowel disease (Fig. 3.19).

Table 3.1 Features that distinguish primary and secondary neoplasms of the colorectum

Feature	Primary neoplasm	Secondary neoplasm
Gross findings		
Single mucosa-based lesion	Common	Common
Multifocal tumor	Uncommon	May be present
Other polyps	May be present	Uncommon
Background of colitis	May be present	Uncommon
Microscopic findings		
Extensive pericolic or serosal tumor deposits	Uncommon	Common
Extensive lymphovascular invasion	Uncommon	May be present
Associated adenoma	Common	Uncommon
Malignant glands with cribriform architecture	Common	Uncommon
Mixed architecture (papillary, acinar, solid)	Uncommon	May be present
Cords of cytologically bland cells	Uncommon	May be present
Dirty necrosis	Common	Uncommon
Solid growth pattern without lymphocytosis	Uncommon	May be present
Small glands with bland cytology	Uncommon	May be present
Nested, trabecular growth	Uncommon	Common
Clear cells	Uncommon	May be present
Psammomatous calcifications	Absent	May be present

Endometriosis

Intestinal endometriosis is a common disease that induces hypertrophy of the muscularis propria in combination with serosal adhesions and may simulate a primary neoplasm. Endometriotic foci are most commonly observed in the outer colonic wall and pericolic soft tissue from the rectosigmoid region (Fig. 3.20). Endometriosis occasionally involves the submucosa and mucosa, where it induces a striking inflammatory response that may

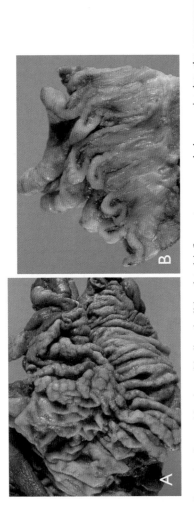

Fig. 3.18 Mural scarring in combination with diverticulitis-related inflammatory mucosal changes simulate the appearance of a colonic carcinoma (**a**). Cross sections of the colon reveal diverticula associated with striking hypertrophy of the muscularis propria and redundancy of mucosal folds (**b**)

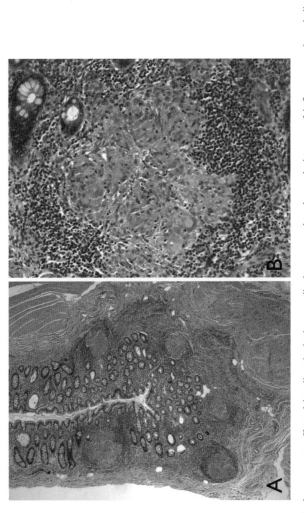

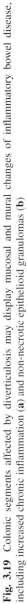

Fig. 3.19 Colonic segments affected by diverticulosis may display mucosal and mural changes of inflammatory bowel disease, including increased chronic inflammation (**a**) and non-necrotic epithelioid granulomas (**b**)

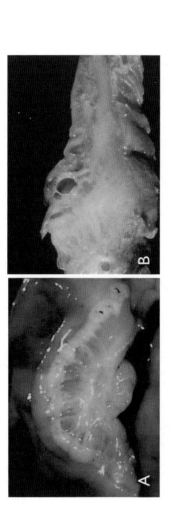

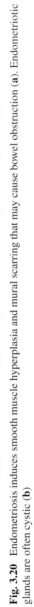

Fig. 3.20 Endometriosis induces smooth muscle hyperplasia and mural scarring that may cause bowel obstruction (**a**). Endometriotic glands are often cystic (**b**)

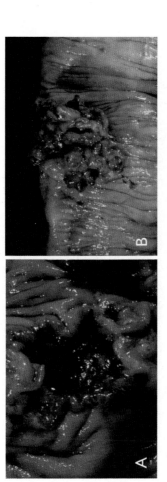

Fig. 3.21 Mural scarring and cystic endometriotic foci may result in mucosal ulceration (**a**) or inflammatory polyps (**b**) that simulate the appearance of colonic cancer

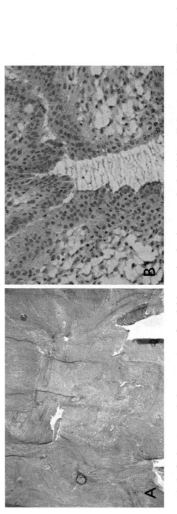

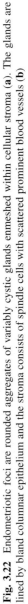

Fig. 3.22 Endometriotic foci are rounded aggregates of variably cystic glands enmeshed within cellular stroma (**a**). The glands are lined by bland columnar epithelium and the stroma consists of spindle cells with scattered prominent blood vessels (**b**)

manifest in the form of inflammatory pseudopolyps or an indurated area of ulceration suspicious for malignancy [4, 5] (Fig. 3.21).

Foci of endometriosis consist of endometrial glands enmeshed within a variable amount of endometriotic stroma with hemorrhage and hemosiderin. Endometriotic deposits appear as well-circumscribed lobules, predominantly in the pericolic tissues and muscularis propria, where they induce inflammation and fibrosis (Fig. 3.22a). The glands are lined by bland columnar epithelium and may be cystically dilated (Fig. 3.22b). Mucosal deposits that colonize the surface epithelium simulate the appearance of epithelial dysplasia [5].

Some patients with colonic endometriosis develop neoplasms of the type observed in the gynecologic tract. Most are endometrioid-type adenocarcinomas, or atypical hyperplasia, although clear cell carcinomas rarely occur. Low-grade endometrial stromal sarcomas and adenosarcomas are much less common. Neoplastic complications of endometriosis may be recognized owing to the spectrum of features observed in most cases and frequent detection of benign foci of endometriosis surrounding the tumor, as previously discussed.

References

1. Michalopoulos A, Papadopoulos V, Zatagias A, et al (2004) Metastatic breast adenocarcinoma masquerading as colonic primary. Report of two cases. Tech Coloproctol 8(Suppl 1):s135–s137
2. Uygun K, Kocak Z, Altaner S, Cicin I, Tokatli F, Uzal C (2006) Colonic metastasis from carcinoma of the breast that mimics a primary intestinal cancer. Yonsei Med J 47(4):578–582
3. McDermott VG, Low VH, Keogan MT, Lawrence JA, Paulson EK (1996) Malignant melanoma metastatic to the gastrointestinal tract. Am J Roentgenol 166(4):809–813
4. Yantiss RK, Clement PB, Young RH (2000) Neoplastic and pre-neoplastic changes in gastrointestinal endometriosis: a study of 17 cases. Am J Surg Pathol 24(4):513–524
5. Yantiss RK, Clement PB, Young RH (2001) Endometriosis of the intestinal tract: a study of 44 cases of a disease that may cause diverse challenges in clinical and pathologic evaluation. Am J Surg Pathol 25(4):445–454

Chapter 4
Non-epithelial Tumors
of the Colorectum

Abstract Several types of mesenchymal and hematopoetic neoplasm may involve the colorectum. Although a definitive diagnosis
is rarely made at the time of frozen section analysis, it is important for the pathologist to be familiar with common mesenchymal
and hematopoetic tumors so that they may facilitate surgical
management and appropriately triage tissue for ancillary studies.
The most common mesenchymal tumors of the colon are gastrointestinal stromal tumors, but neoplasms that recapitulate the
phenotypes of smooth muscle cells, Schwann cells, and fibroblasts
also develop in this location. Most hematopoetic neoplasms that
involve the colon are B-cell lymphomas, and they may affect either
immunocompetent or immunocompromised individuals.

Keywords Gastrointestinal stromal tumor · Fibromatosis ·
Lymphoma

Introduction

The majority of malignant colonic tumors are epithelial carcinomas, although mesenchymal tumors and lymphomas may occur as
primary, or secondary, malignancies. Most mesenchymal tumors
are situated in the muscularis propria, or outer colonic wall,

N.C. Panarelli, R.K. Yantiss, *Frozen Section Library: Appendix,*
Colon, and Anus, Frozen Section Library 4, DOI 10.1007/978-1-4419-6584-4_4,
© Springer Science+Business Media, LLC 2010

and are not amenable to colonoscopic biopsy, whereas hemato-
logic malignancies closely simulate the radiographic and clinical
appearance of colorectal carcinoma. Although a definitive diagnosis may not be required at the time of frozen section, pathologists
should be familiar with the features of common mesenchymal and
hematopoetic neoplasms, so they may guide the surgical management of the patient and appropriately triage tissue for subsequent
ancillary studies.

Mesenchymal Lesions

Gastrointestinal Stromal Tumor

Most surgically removed mesenchymal tumors that affect the colon
are either gastrointestinal stromal tumors or intra-abdominal fibromatoses, although a variety of other lesions may be infrequently
encountered (Table 4.1). The distinction between different types of
sarcoma at the time of frozen section is generally unnecessary, but
a diagnosis of intra-abdominal fibromatosis should be suggested in
the appropriate context, since extensive surgical resection of these
benign, but locally aggressive, tumors may result in substantial
patient morbidity. Gastrointestinal stromal tumors occur in any age
group but are most common among older adults. The epicenter of
the tumor lies within the muscularis propria, presumably because
these lesions recapitulate the phenotype of interstitial cells of Cajal
that reside in, or near, the myenteric plexus. Most colorectal gastrointestinal stromal tumors are large, bulky tumors with a fleshy
cut surface and may display cystic degeneration, hemorrhage, or
necrosis (Fig. 4.1). They are usually quite cellular and contain
predominantly spindle cells with abundant eosinophilic cytoplasm
and minimal cytologic atypia (Fig. 4.2). Gastrointestinal stromal
tumors show a greater degree of cellularity than leiomyomas, the
latter of which are usually small, polypoid lesions derived from
the muscularis mucosae, whereas large leiomyomas derived from
the muscularis propria are quite rare (Fig. 4.3). On the other

Table 4.1 Mesenchymal tumors of the colorectum

Tumor	Epicenter location	Patients affected
Gastrointestinal stromal tumor	Muscularis propria	Older adults, neurofibromatosis
Smooth muscle neoplasms		
Leiomyoma	Muscularis mucosae	Incidental at endoscopy
Leiomyosarcoma	Muscularis propria	Older adults
EBV-associated smooth muscle tumors	Muscularis propria	Immunosuppressed patients
Nerve sheath tumors		
Schwannoma	Muscularis propria	Adults
Neurofibroma	Diffuse in wall	Neurofibromatosis
Perineuroma	Mucosa	Incidental at endoscopy
Granular cell tumor	Usually superficial	Adults
Malignant peripheral nerve sheath tumor	Outer wall/ mesentery	Older adults
Fibroblastic lesions		
Mesenteric fibromatosis	Outer wall/ mesentery	Young adults, Gardner's syndrome
Inflammatory myofibroblastic tumor	Outer wall/ mesentery	Children, young adults
Sclerosing mesenteritis	Outer wall/ mesentery	Adults, some IgG4-mediated

hand, leiomyosarcomas display overtly malignant cytologic features compared to gastrointestinal stromal tumors [1] (Fig. 4.4). One should defer subclassification of malignant mesenchymal neoplasms and gastrointestinal stromal tumors until full review of the permanent tissue sections, since the biologic risk of the latter is related to tumor size and mitotic activity, as enumerated in Table 4.2 [2].

Intra-abdominal Fibromatosis

Mesenteric fibromatosis is a neoplastic proliferation of fibroblasts within mesenteric fat that secondarily involves the colonic

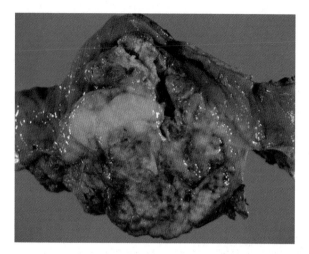

Fig. 4.1 This colonic gastrointestinal stromal tumor undermines the mucosa, forming a fungating, ulcerated mass, although most of the tumor lies in the colonic wall and pericolic soft tissues. The cut surface is heterogeneous with areas of hemorrhage and necrosis

wall. Although this type of tumor has no capacity for metastasis, it is locally aggressive and may encroach upon vital structures, such as blood vessels and the tubular gut. Fibromatoses occur more commonly among young adults (<40 years of age) and may represent a manifestation of some gastrointestinal polyposis disorders. The tumors have an infiltrative appearance and firm, gray, homogeneous cut surface (Fig. 4.5). They contain sweeping fascicles of spindled fibroblasts with fine, delicate cytoplasm and bland nuclei enmeshed within variably collagenous stroma (Fig. 4.6). Thick-walled blood vessels and perivascular hemorrhage are commonly encountered (Fig. 4.7). Fibromatoses may display relatively frequent mitotic figures, but this finding should not be considered reflective of their biologic potential. Fibromatoses are generally more cellular than non-neoplastic fibroproliferative lesions, such as sclerosing mesenteritis [3] (Fig. 4.8).

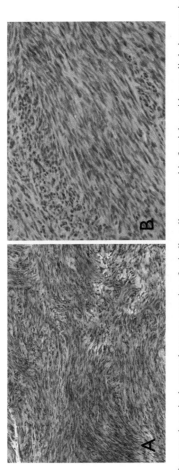

Fig. 4.2 Colonic gastrointestinal stromal tumors consist of spindle cells arranged in fascicles with very little intervening stroma (**a**). The cells contain abundant eosinophilic cytoplasm and elongated, but cytologically bland, nuclei (**b**)

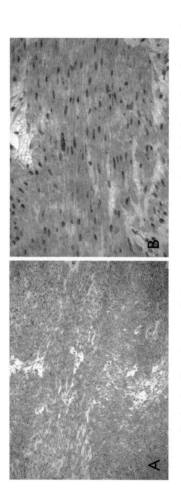

Fig. 4.3 Leiomyomas usually develop from the muscularis mucosae, so most are detected during endoscopic procedures. They are less cellular than gastrointestinal stromal tumors and consist of spindle cells arranged in sweeping fascicles that intersect at 90° angles (**a**). The tumor cells contain abundant, brightly eosinophilic cytoplasm and elongated nuclei with minimal cytologic atypia and virtually no mitotic activity (**b**)

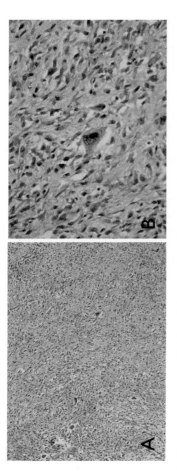

Fig. 4.4 Colonic leiomyosarcomas are highly cellular, overtly malignant neoplasms comprised of variable numbers of spindle and epithelioid cells (**a**). The cells contain ample eosinophilic cytoplasm and display severely atypical cytologic features with large, hyperchromatic nuclei and easily identifiable mitotic figures (**b**)

Table 4.2 Risk stratification of gastrointestinal stromal tumors

Predicted risk	Size	Mitoses
Very low risk	<2 cm	<5/50 high-power fields (hpf)
Low risk	2–5 cm	<5/50 hpf
Intermediate risk	<5 cm 5–10 cm	6–10/50 hpf <5/50 hpf
High risk	>5 cm >10 cm Any size	>5/50 hpf Any mitotic rate >10/50 hpf

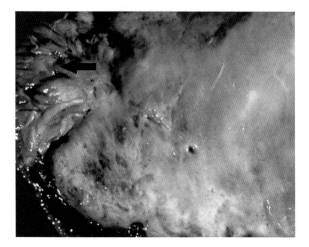

Fig. 4.5 Mesenteric fibromatosis is a large soft tissue mass that infiltrates the bowel wall (*arrow*). The tumor is ill-defined with a firm, or gritty, *gray-white* cut surface

Hematopoetic Neoplasms

Most colonic lymphomas are B-cell neoplasms (Table 4.3). Primary T-cell and NK-cell lymphomas occur in the colon but are exceedingly rare. Low-grade tumors may develop in otherwise healthy patients, whereas immunosuppressed patients and those with inflammatory bowel disease are at risk for high-grade lesions [4, 5]. Intraoperative evaluation should include a combination of frozen sections and touch preparations to evaluate architecture and

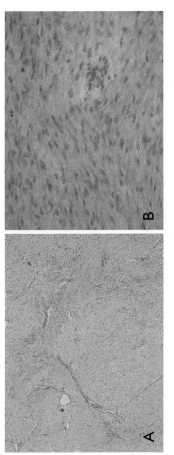

Fig. 4.6 Intra-abdominal fibromatosis consists of long, sweeping fascicles of spindle cells enmeshed within a variably collagenous stroma (**a**). The spindle cells contain faintly eosinophilic, tapering cytoplasmic processes and ovoid to elongated nuclei with even chromatin and small, but conspicuous, nucleoli (**b**)

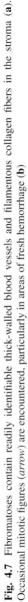

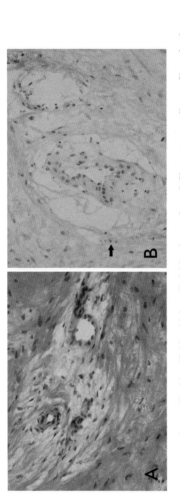

Fig. 4.7 Fibromatoses contain readily identifiable thick-walled blood vessels and filamentous collagen fibers in the stroma (**a**). Occasional mitotic figures (*arrow*) are encountered, particularly in areas of fresh hemorrhage (**b**)

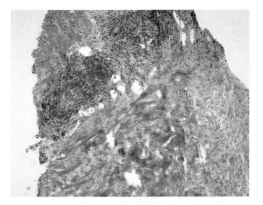

Fig. 4.8 Sclerosing mesenteritis is a poorly characterized inflammatory process that may involve the colon. The tumors contain fibroblasts enmeshed within collagenous stroma, often in combination with mononuclear cell rich inflammation

Table 4.3 Pathologic features of primary B-cell lymphomas of the colon

Diffuse large B cell lymphoma	Architecture: sheets of cells infiltrate between crypts
	Cytology: large cells, vesicular chromatin, multiple nucleoli, abundant cytoplasm
MALT lymphoma	Architecture: neoplastic cells in mantle zone and overrun follicles, lymphoepithelial lesions
	Cytology: plasma cells and centrocyte-like cells with irregular nuclei, inconspicuous nucleoli, pale cytoplasm
Mantle cell lymphoma (lymphomatous polyposis)	Architecture: multiple intestinal polyps comprised of lymphoid nodules with "naked" germinal centers trapped within neoplastic mantle zone
	Cytology: small-to-medium cells with irregular nuclei resembling centrocytes
Follicular lymphoma	Architecture: uniform lymphoid follicles with compressed intervening stroma that lack polarity and tingible body macrophages
	Cytology: predominantly centrocytes in most cases
Burkitt lymphoma	Architecture: sheets of blasts with interspersed histiocytes
	Cytology: clumped chromatin, multiple basophilic nucleoli, thin rim of cytoplasm

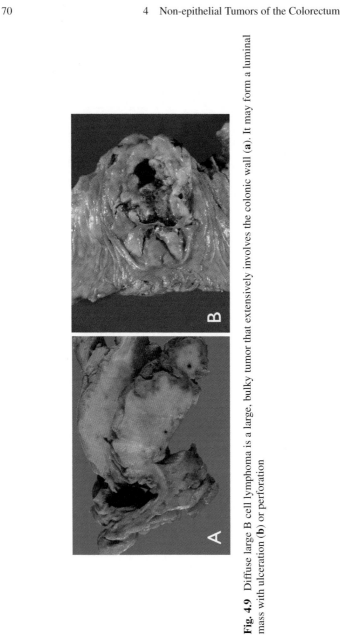

Fig. 4.9 Diffuse large B cell lymphoma is a large, bulky tumor that extensively involves the colonic wall (**a**). It may form a luminal mass with ulceration (**b**) or perforation

cytology. Specific diagnoses are deferred to permanent sections and ancillary studies, but priority should be placed on establishing the hematopoetic nature of the neoplasm to ensure that tissue is triaged for flow cytometry, cytogenetics, and immunohistochemistry appropriately.

Although low-grade B cell lymphomas affect the colon more commonly than high-grade tumors, diffuse large B cell lymphoma is the most likely high-grade lymphoma to produce a bulky mass requiring intraoperative consultation [6]. Diffuse large B cell lymphomas may arise de novo or reflect high-grade transformation of extranodal marginal zone lymphoma of mucosa-associated lymphoid tissue (MALT lymphoma) [4–7]. Most high-grade lymphomas are infiltrative lesions that produce mural and mucosal thickening with or without ulceration and simulate the appearance of colonic carcinoma (Fig. 4.9). Tumor cells contain relatively scant cytoplasm with large round nuclei that display heterogeneous chromatin and one, or more, nucleoli (Fig. 4.10). Burkitt-type lymphomas show a predilection for the proximal colon, particularly

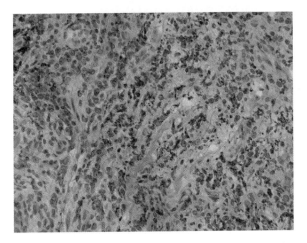

Fig. 4.10 Neoplastic B cells permeate the colonic wall in sheets. The tumor cells contain a variable amount of eosinophilic cytoplasm and large, round nuclei with peripherally condensed chromatin and prominent nucleoli. Single necrotic tumor cells and mitotic figures are readily apparent

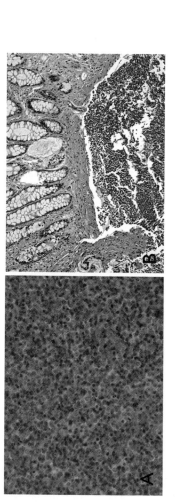
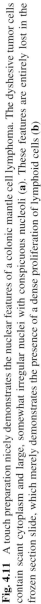

Fig. 4.11 A touch preparation nicely demonstrates the nuclear features of a colonic mantle cell lymphoma. The dyshesive tumor cells contain scant cytoplasm and large, somewhat irregular nuclei with conspicuous nucleoli (**a**). These features are entirely lost in the frozen section slide, which merely demonstrates the presence of a dense proliferation of lymphoid cells (**b**)

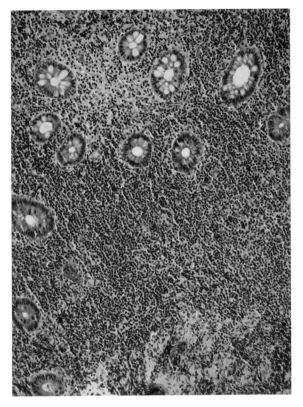

Fig. 4.12 Low-grade follicular lymphoma diffusely involves the mucosa and submucosa. Unlike reactive inflammatory processes, including colitis, the infiltrate is similarly dense at all levels in the mucosa, and neutrophilic inflammation is lacking

the ileocecal region [5]. Most high-grade lymphomas show overtly malignant features, so the main differential diagnosis includes primary, or metastatic, carcinoma and metastatic melanoma. A diagnosis of lymphoma may be suspected owing to the complete lack of gland formation, as would be expected of virtually all colorectal carcinomas, as well as the presence of extensive transmural involvement of the colon and absence of a mucosal epithelial

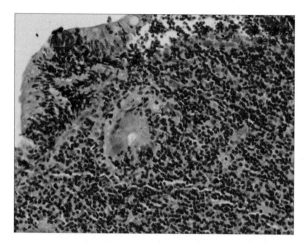

Fig. 4.13 Low-grade extranodal marginal zone (MALT) lymphoma cells permeate the mucosa and infiltrate colonic crypts (lymphoepithelial lesions)

neoplasm. Touch preparations are extremely useful, since they demonstrate fine nuclear detail, which is not appreciable in most frozen sections (Fig. 4.11).

Distinguishing between low-grade lymphoma and normal lymphoid tissue of the colorectum may be problematic, since abundant lymphoid tissue is normally present in both the proximal colon and rectum. Low-grade lymphomas commonly manifest as mucosal, or submucosal, nodules resulting from expansion of preexisting lymphoid follicles, thereby simulating the appearance of colorectal polyps. The lymphoid cells diffusely permeate the mucosa between the colonic crypts, and the infiltrate is similarly dense at all levels in the mucosa (Fig. 4.12). Crypt destruction by clusters of lymphoid cells is not typical of most forms of colitis, so its presence in combination with dense lymphoid inflammation should raise concern for a neoplasm (Fig. 4.13). Mantle cell and follicular lymphomas classically appear as innumerable polyps that simulate the appearance of a heritable disorder and, indeed, this finding has been termed "lymphomatoid polyposis" (Fig. 4.14) [7].

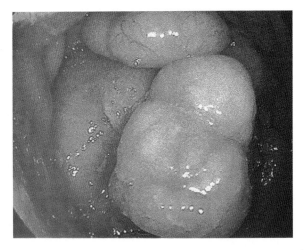

Fig. 4.14 Mantle cell lymphoma expands preexisting mucosa-associated lymphoid tissue in the colon, producing innumerable polyps

References

1. Fenoglio-Preiser CM, Noffsinger AE, Stemmermann GN, Lantz PE, Isaacson PG (2008) Mesenchymal tumors. Gastrointestinal pathology: an atlas and text. Lippincott Williams & Wilkins, Philadelphia, PA, pp 1203–1265
2. Fletcher CDM, Berman JJ, Corless C, et al (2002) Diagnosis of gastrointestinal stromal tumors: a consensus approach. Hum Pathol 33:459–465
3. Mathew J, McKenna F, Mason J, Haboubi NY, Borghol M (2004) Sclerosing mesenteritis with occult ileal perforation: report of a case simulating extensive intra-abdominal malignancy. Dis Colon Rectum 47(11):1974–1977
4. Dionigi G, Annoni M, Rovera F, et al (2007) Primary colorectal lymphomas: review of the literature. Surg Oncol 16(Suppl 1):s169–s171
5. Wong MT, Eu KW (2006) Primary colorectal lymphomas. Colorectal Dis 8(7):586–591
6. Gonzalez QH, Heslin MJ, Davila-Cervantes A, et al (2008) Primary colonic lymphoma. Am Surg 74(3):214–216
7. Li B, Shi YK, He XH, et al (2008) Primary non-Hodgkin lymphomas of the small and large intestine: clinicopathological characteristics and management of 40 patients. Int J Hematol 87(4):375–381

Chapter 5
Frozen Section Assessment of the Colorectum in the Pediatric Population

Abstract The most common indication for intraoperative consultation among pediatric patients with gastrointestinal symptoms is evaluation for the possibility of Hirschsprung's disease. Intraoperative documentation of ganglion cells, or their absence, is crucial to the immediate management of the patient. Unfortunately, detecting ganglion cells in colonic samples obtained from neonatal patients may be challenging for a number of reasons, not the least of which is their immature appearance in frozen section samples.

Keywords Hirschsprung's disease · Hypoganglionosis · Intestinal neuronal dysplasia · Ganglion cell · Motility

Introduction

Evaluation of gastrointestinal motility disorders is one of the most frequent indications for intraoperative consultation among pediatric patients with gastrointestinal symptoms; yet assessment for Hirschsprung's disease is one of the most challenging situations encountered in the frozen section laboratory. Pathologists need to be aware of the diagnostic features and potential pitfalls encountered when dealing with colorectal samples obtained from pediatric patients.

N.C. Panarelli, R.K. Yantiss, *Frozen Section Library: Appendix,*
Colon, and Anus, Frozen Section Library 4, DOI 10.1007/978-1-4419-6584-4_5,
© Springer Science+Business Media, LLC 2010

Hirschsprung's Disease

Hirschsprung's disease is a congenital condition defined by the lack of parasympathetic ganglion cells in the intramural and submucosal plexuses, which results in inadequate propulsive movement and constipation. The disease affects the colon in a retrograde fashion, such that ganglion cells are always lacking in the distal colorectum, but may be present more proximally [1]. Total colonic aganglionosis also occurs, although rarely. Management of Hirschsprung's disease is variable. At some institutions, patients with suspected Hirschsprung's disease undergo endoscopic mucosal suction biopsy of the distal 2–3 cm of rectum, as well as sampling of more proximal colon. If these samples contain adequate submucosa to assess for the presence of ganglion cells, then clinicians will be aware of the location of the transition area prior to surgery. Individuals who lack ganglion cells in endoscopically obtained material are subjected to surgery that requires intraoperative frozen section evaluation. Full-thickness biopsies obtained from the distal colorectum, transition between dilated and normal caliber colonic segments, and site of imminent colostomy are assessed intraoperatively by frozen section analysis for the presence of ganglion cells. Procurement of tissue samples is followed by creation of a colostomy and closure. A second surgical procedure follows detection of the transition area, during which the aganglionic segment is removed and a colo-anal pull-through anastomosis is created [1]. Alternatively, anastomosis of the normally innervated colon to the anus is performed immediately upon identification of the transition area by frozen section analysis [1]. Therefore, surgeons rely heavily upon pathologists for accurate identification of normally innervated bowel, and discrepancies between interpretations of frozen and permanent sections have important clinical implications. Failure to recognize ganglion cells that are present results in unnecessarily extensive resection, whereas misclassification of other cell types as ganglion cells necessitates a second operation [1].

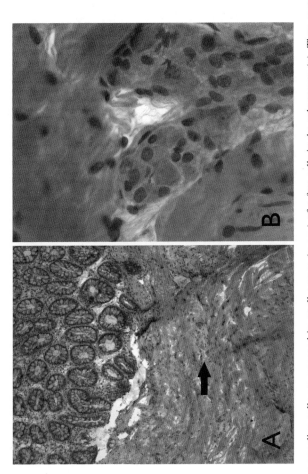

Fig. 5.1 Mature ganglion cells are arranged in small groups (*arrow*) of a few cells in the submucosa (**a**). They contain abundant cytoplasm and large nuclei with nucleoli (**b**)

Ganglion cells are large, polygonal cells with abundant eosinophilic cytoplasm, round nuclei, and prominent nucleoli. They are frequently arranged in clusters within the submucosa (Meissner's plexus) and may be accompanied by small nerve fibers (Fig. 5.1). Ganglion cells are more numerous and readily identifiable in the myenteric plexus (Fig. 5.2). However, they are immature during the neonatal period and contain less cytoplasm, smaller nuclei, and inconspicuous nucleoli (Fig. 5.3). In this situation, they may not be readily identifiable owing to severe freezing artifact, or superficial sectioning at the time of frozen section, so multiple serial sections may aid their detection [1]. One should also note that the distal-most aspect of the rectum (distal 1–2 cm) is hypoganglionic, or aganglionic, and that samples of this area may fail to reveal ganglion cells. Thus, samples that contain squamous (anal) mucosa normally lack ganglion cells, and failure to recognize them in biopsies from the anorectal junction should not be taken as evidence of Hirschsprung's disease. Most, if not all, cases of Hirschsprung's disease display proliferating nerve fibers in the submucosa and muscularis propria in addition to an absence of ganglion cells (Fig. 5.4).

Hypoganglionosis

Hypoganglionosis is defined as decreased numbers of ganglion cells (<14/cm) as well as diminished nuclear diameter in ganglion cells of the affected colon relative to those in the normally innervated bowel [2]. It is commonly encountered in colonic segments proximal to the transition area in patients with Hirschsprung's disease, so pathologists should probably limit their comments to the presence, or absence, of ganglion cells, rather than their numbers, when analysis is limited to a biopsy sample [1]. Comments regarding the adequacy of innervation should be confined to situations in which the pathologist has access to the entire circumference of the colon, in order to estimate the volume of ganglion cells present. Surgical anastomosis to a hypoganglionic colonic segment

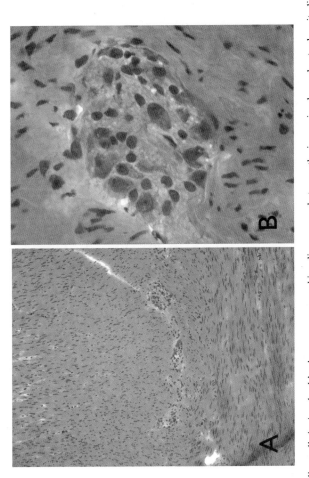

Fig. 5.2 Ganglion cells in Auerbach's plexus are arranged in a linear array between the inner circular and outer longitudinal layers of the muscularis propria (**a**) and tend to be grouped in large clusters (**b**)

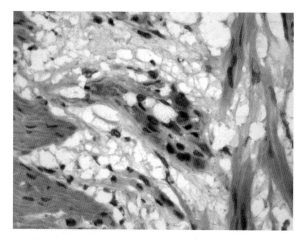

Fig. 5.3 Colonic samples obtained during the neonatal period contain immature-appearing ganglion cells with relatively scant cytoplasm, small nuclei, and inconspicuous nucleoli

may result in persistent symptoms in patients with Hirschsprung's disease [1].

Intestinal Neuronal Dysplasia

Intestinal neuronal dysplasia is an umbrella term that describes a heterogeneous group of motility disorders characterized by clinical symptoms of constipation, despite the presence of ganglion cells. The clinicopathologic features of this entity have not been well defined, but colons from some patients have a hypertrophic, band-like myenteric plexus that contains "giant" ganglia consisting of groups of more than eight ganglion cells, as well as isolated ganglion cells in the submucosa and mucosa [3]. Frozen sections are not performed to evaluate for the presence of intestinal neuronal dysplasia, but fresh samples may be frozen in order to perform special histochemical stains, such as acetylcholine esterase.

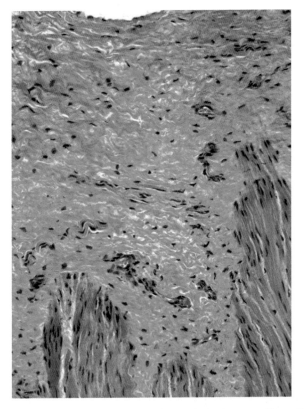

Fig. 5.4 Patients with Hirschsprung's disease do not have ganglion cells in the mucosa or submucosa of the affected colonic segment. However, a lack of ganglion cells is usually accompanied by hyperplasia and hypertrophy of nerves in the submucosa

References

1. Shayan K, Smith C, Langer JC (2004) Reliability of intraoperative frozen section in the management of Hirschsprung's disease. J Pediatr Surg 39(9):1345–1348
2. Tagushi T, Masumoto K, Ieiri S, Nakatsuji T, Akiyoshi J (2006) New classification of hypoganglionosis: congenital and acquired hypoganglionosis. J Pediatr Surg 41(12):2046–2051

3. Kobayashi H, Hirakawa H, Surana R, O'Brian SD, Puri P (1995) Intestinal neuronal dysplasia is a possible cause of persistent bowel symptoms after pull-through operation for Hirschsprung's disease. J Pediatr Surg 30(2):253–259

Chapter 6
Frozen Section Evaluation
of the Appendix

Abstract Appendiceal tumors are rarely diagnosed preoperatively, and their classification is both challenging and controversial
owing to their tendency to disseminate in the peritoneal cavity
despite their frequent low-grade appearance. Frozen section analysis may be requested to assess the status of the appendiceal margin,
determine whether extra-appendiceal epithelium is present, and to
classify extra-appendiceal disease as low- or high-grade. Other
types of appendiceal epithelial tumors, such as serrated neoplasms, should be distinguished from mucinous tumors, since
they tend to precede overtly malignant peritoneal disease (peritoneal carcinomatosis). Goblet cell carcinoid tumors often spread
to non-contiguous structures and, thus, may prompt intraoperative
consultation.

Keywords Appendicitis · Mucinous neoplasm · Extra-appendiceal
mucin · Endocrine · Goblet cell carcinoid

Introduction

Primary appendiceal tumors are found in less than 2% of surgically removed appendices and typically bear a resemblance to
their colonic counterparts. Most epithelial tumors are mucinous or
contain villous projections, and those with serrated architecture

N.C. Panarelli, R.K. Yantiss, *Frozen Section Library: Appendix,*
Colon, and Anus, Frozen Section Library 4, DOI 10.1007/978-1-4419-6584-4_6,
© Springer Science+Business Media, LLC 2010

are increasingly recognized. Appendiceal endocrine neoplasms are relatively common, incidentally discovered lesions that generally do not require intraoperative consultation, although goblet cell "carcinoid" tumors may pose challenges to both surgeons and pathologists [1]. Unfortunately, the diagnosis of appendiceal neoplasia is rarely made preoperatively, since many patients have clinical symptoms of appendicitis [2, 3]. As a result, intraoperative frozen section evaluation is commonly performed to determine the surgical management of patients with these tumors. Most important issues revolve around the diagnosis and classification of mucinous neoplasms, as discussed below.

Appendicitis

The acutely inflamed appendix displays serosal hyperemia with or without fibrinopurulent exudates and inflammation (Fig. 6.1). Mucosal necrosis is accompanied by purulent luminal debris and neutrophilic inflammation within the muscularis propria, which

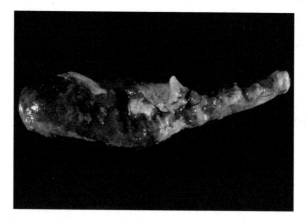

Fig. 6.1 An acutely inflamed appendix displays fibrinous adhesions on the erythematous serosa. Inflammation in the mesoappendiceal fat reflects perforation and a periappendiceal abscess

may be associated with mesoappendiceal abscesses. A prolonged interval between the onset of symptoms and surgical resection may result in intense eosinophil-rich inflammation in combination with granulomas, a foreign body giant cell-rich response to luminal material, and organizing serositis (Fig. 6.2). Sheets of tissue macrophages laden with ceroid pigment in combination with multinucleated giant cells and fat necrosis may prompt a diagnosis of "xanthogranulomatous appendicitis".

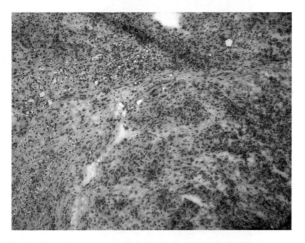

Fig. 6.2 Prolonged acute appendicitis produces a fibroinflammatory appendiceal mass that simulates a neoplasm. One may observe a mixed inflammatory cell infiltrate with sheets of macrophages associated with fat necrosis and fibrosis

Appendiceal Mucinous Neoplasms

Epithelial neoplasms of the appendix are generally classified as mucinous neoplasms and non-mucinous tumors. Appendiceal mucinous neoplasms characteristically cause cystic dilatation of the appendix, but they may rupture, resulting in accumulation of mucin around the appendix (Fig. 6.3). Mucinous appendiceal neoplasms may also disseminate through the peritoneum in the

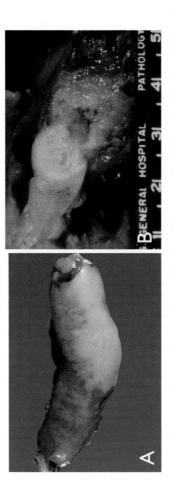
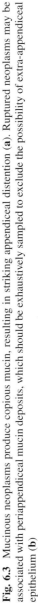

Fig. 6.3 Mucinous neoplasms produce copious mucin, resulting in striking appendiceal distention (**a**). Ruptured neoplasms may be associated with periappendiceal mucin deposits, which should be exhaustively sampled to exclude the possibility of extra-appendiceal epithelium (**b**)

form of mucin deposits, or pseudomyxoma peritonei (Fig. 6.4). They frequently metastasize to the ovary, which may be large and cystic, simulating the appearance of a primary ovarian neoplasm (Figs. 6.5 and 6.6). Pathologists will be called upon to classify peritoneal tumor deposits in many institutions because immediate treatment depends upon the degree of atypia present in extra-appendiceal epithelium. Patients with low-grade peritoneal disease may be treated with surgical debulking and peritoneal stripping with the aim of complete cytoreduction either with, or without, intraoperative intraperitoneal chemotherapy. Moderate-to-poorly differentiated mucinous carcinomas may also produce gelatinous ascites, but they do not respond to cytoreductive surgery, so these patients may be offered systemic chemotherapy. Therefore, pathologists should clearly communicate the histologic findings and biologic implications of their observations at the time of the frozen section.

Mucinous lesions typically display a circumferential growth pattern in the appendiceal mucosa and contain tall columnar mucinous cells arranged in a single layer, or papillae with low-grade nuclei [4] (Fig. 6.7). When present, extra-appendiceal disease consists of pools of mucin containing strips or clusters of neoplastic epithelial cells that usually show bland cytologic features, similar to those of the appendiceal component [5] (Fig. 6.8).

Several groups have proposed a variety of classification schemes that employ varied, and often confusing, terminology to describe appendiceal mucinous tumors [6–10] (Table 6.1). Most studies have shown that mucinous neoplasia confined to the appendiceal mucosa is essentially cured by excision, regardless of the degree of dysplasia, whereas peritoneal disease is associated with disease recurrence and death in nearly half of patients. Emerging data also suggest that acellular mucin pools limited to the appendiceal wall and periappendix are associated with an excellent prognosis, provided the entire appendix is submitted for histologic evaluation to exclude the possibility of extra-appendiceal epithelium. However, any amount of extra-appendiceal epithelium may be associated with progressive mucinous ascites and death in some cases, even if one identifies only rare clusters of neoplastic epithelial cells surrounding the appendix [5] (Fig. 6.9). Extension

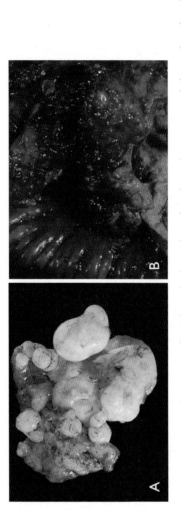

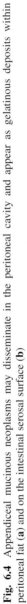

Fig. 6.4 Appendiceal mucinous neoplasms may disseminate in the peritoneal cavity and appear as gelatinous deposits within peritoneal fat (**a**) and on the intestinal serosal surface (**b**)

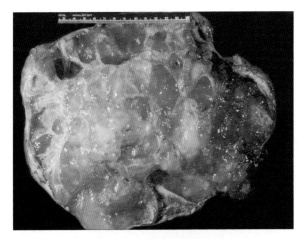

Fig. 6.5 Metastatic appendiceal mucinous tumors result in massive ovarian enlargement with multiple loculated cysts filled with mucinous material

beyond the appendix should also be distinguished from herniations of mucosa through the wall, or diverticula, since this finding has no biologic implications (Fig. 6.10).

The proposed classification schemes for appendiceal mucinous neoplasia reflect differences of opinion regarding the fundamental nature of peritoneal disease. At one extreme, some investigators feel that peritoneal dissemination results from appendiceal rupture and spillage of both mucin and neoplastic, but non-invasive, epithelium into the peritoneal cavity. Proponents of this hypothesis classify tumors limited to the appendiceal mucosa as mucinous cystadenomas. They consider gelatinous ascites containing low-grade epithelium to represent disseminated peritoneal adenomucinosis but reserve the term "carcinoma" for tumors that display high-grade cytologic features (Figs. 6.11 and 6.12) [8, 10]. Conversely, most authorities, including the World Health Organization, now consider pseudomyxoma peritonei to represent carcinoma and grade the cytologic features present in extra-appendiceal epithelium. Low-grade tumors corresponding to "disseminated peritoneal adenomucinosis" are classified as low-grade

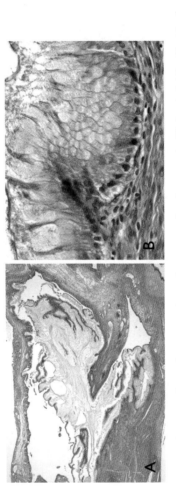

Fig. 6.6 Appendiceal mucinous neoplasms that metastasize to the ovary produce large mucin-filled cysts (**a**) lined by bland epithelium that may simulate a primary ovarian tumor (**b**)

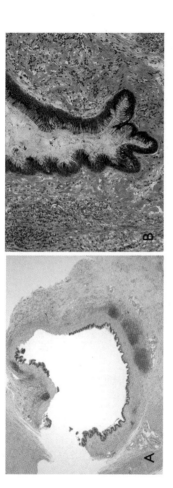

Fig. 6.7 Mucinous neoplasms circumferentially involve the appendiceal mucosa (**a**) and contain villous, or flat, low-grade mucinous epithelium with slightly enlarged, basally located nuclei (**b**)

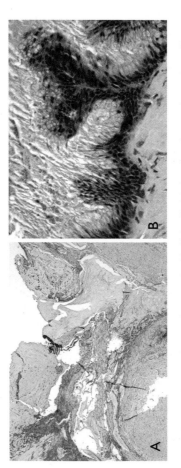

Fig. 6.8 Peritoneal mucin deposits contain rare clusters of epithelial cells (**a**) that show low-grade cytology (**b**)

Table 6.1 Proposed classification schemes for appendiceal mucinous neoplasms

	Carr and Sobin	Misdraji et al.	Pai and Longacre	Ronnett et al.	World Health Organization
Tumor confined to appendix					
Limited to mucosa					
Low-grade cytology	Adenoma	Low-grade appendiceal mucinous neoplasm	Adenoma	Adenoma	Adenoma
High-grade cytology	Adenoma	Non-invasive mucinous cystadenocarcinoma	Adenoma	Adenoma	Adenoma
Positive surgical margin	Adenoma	Low-grade appendiceal mucinous neoplasm	Uncertain malignant potential		Adenoma
Cellular mucin in wall	Invasive mucinous adenocarcinoma	Low-grade appendiceal mucinous neoplasm	Uncertain malignant potential		Invasive mucinous adenocarcinoma
Tumor beyond appendix					
Low-grade epithelium in peritoneal mucin	Invasive mucinous adenocarcinoma	Low-grade appendiceal mucinous neoplasm	Low-grade with high risk of recurrence	Disseminated peritoneal adenomucinosis	Low-grade mucinous adenocarcinoma
High-grade epithelium in peritoneal mucin	Invasive mucinous adenocarcinoma	Invasive mucinous adenocarcinoma	Invasive mucinous adenocarcinoma	Peritoneal mucinous carcinomatosis	High-grade mucinous adenocarcinoma

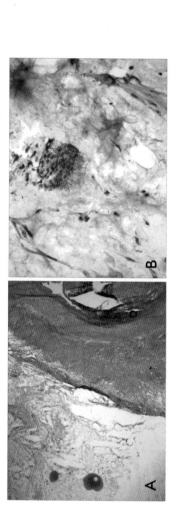
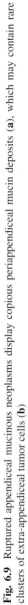

Fig. 6.9 Ruptured appendiceal mucinous neoplasms display copious periappendiceal mucin deposits (**a**), which may contain rare clusters of extra-appendiceal tumor cells (**b**)

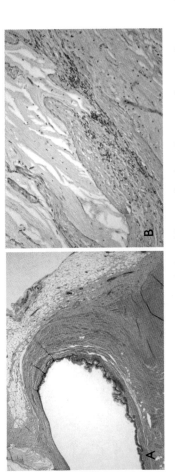

Fig. 6.10 Diverticula are commonly encountered in association with appendiceal mucinous neoplasms and represent herniations of mucosa through the muscularis propria (**a**). Ruptured diverticula may be associated with acellular organizing mucin in the mesoappendix and on the serosa but should not be interpreted to represent a neoplasm (**b**)

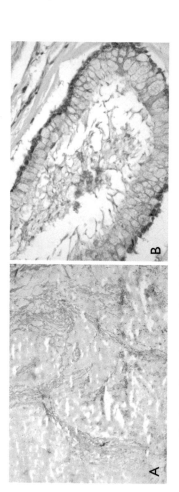

Fig. 6.11 Mucinous appendiceal neoplasms that spread to the peritoneal cavity should be classified based on the degree of cytologic atypia present in extra-appendiceal epithelium. Low-grade lesions consist of mucin pools (**a**) that contain scant strips or clusters of mucinous epithelium with minimal cytologic atypia (**b**). These lesions are considered to represent disseminated peritoneal adenomucinosis by some and low-grade mucinous adenocarcinoma by others

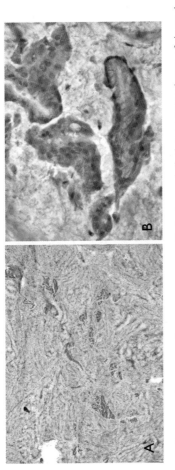

Fig. 6.12 Some mucinous neoplasms contain more numerous cell clusters and display a greater degree of tissue destruction and invasion (**a**). These lesions typically show severely atypical cytologic features with enlarged, round nuclei, nucleoli, and mitotic figures (**b**). Peritoneal involvement pursues an aggressive course, does not respond well to surgical debulking, and should be classified as adenocarcinoma

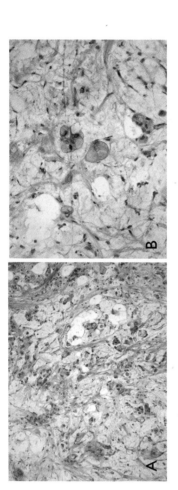

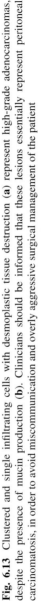

Fig. 6.13 Clustered and single infiltrating cells with desmoplastic tissue destruction (**a**) represent high-grade adenocarcinomas, despite the presence of mucin production (**b**). Clinicians should be informed that these lesions essentially represent peritoneal carcinomatosis, in order to avoid miscommunication and overly aggressive surgical management of the patient

mucinous adenocarcinomas (Figs. 6.8, 6.9, and 6.11). More cellular lesions that display malignant cytology are considered to represent high-grade mucinous adenocarcinomas [5, 11] (Fig. 6.12). Notably, carcinomas that infiltrate the peritoneal soft tissue as single cells or cluster associated with desmoplasia are uniformly classified as high-grade adenocarcinomas, regardless of the presence of mucin production. They seed the peritoneum in the form of solid tumor nodules, or carcinomatosis, which is not amenable to surgery (Fig. 6.13). The term "mucinous adenocarcinoma" is generally avoided when describing such cancers in order to avoid confusion.

The primary goals of intraoperative examination are to (1) determine whether the mucinous neoplasm is limited to the appendix, (2) assess extra-appendiceal mucin for the presence of neoplastic epithelium, and (3) grade the severity of cytologic atypia within extra-appendiceal epithelium. Tumors limited to the appendix are treated with appendectomy alone, whereas a right colectomy or cecectomy may be considered when the appendix is ruptured, or the neoplasm is present at the appendiceal resection margin.

Non-mucinous Appendiceal Epithelial Neoplasms

Non-mucinous adenomas and carcinomas are histologically similar to their colonic counterparts and are commonly referred to as "colonic-type" lesions (Fig. 6.14). Colonic-type appendiceal adenomas are relatively uncommon and are generally observed in patients with familial adenomatous polyposis or represent colonic adenomas that extend to involve the appendiceal mucosa from the cecum [4]. More frequently, non-mucinous appendiceal neoplasms display serrated architecture. They may contain non-dysplastic or dysplastic epithelium and show molecular features similar to those of serrated colonic polyps [12] (Fig. 6.15).

Serrated appendiceal lesions are relatively common, but have been poorly characterized. They are usually incidentally discovered in colectomy specimens obtained for medical indications but

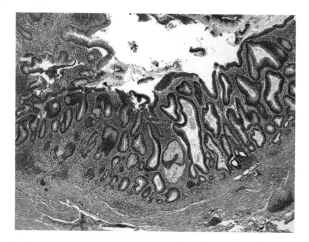

Fig. 6.14 Colonic-type appendiceal adenomas protrude into the lumen and contain cells with enlarged pseudostratified nuclei and faintly eosinophilic cytoplasm, reminiscent of tubular or villous adenomas of the colon

may occur in patients with concomitant proximal colon cancers. Importantly, serrated appendiceal lesions occasionally precede invasive adenocarcinomas that show overtly malignant features and a destructive growth pattern characteristic of colonic cancers (Fig. 6.16a). Although these cancers may contain abundant extracellular mucin, peritoneal disease is in the form of solid tumor nodules, and pursues a uniformly malignant course (Fig. 6.16b). Therefore, this type of tumor should not be considered within the spectrum of pseudomyxoma peritonei but is simply graded and staged as invasive adenocarcinoma [12].

Endocrine Neoplasms of the Appendix

The most common appendiceal tumors are well-differentiated endocrine neoplasms. These tumors have been historically classified as "carcinoid" tumors because they are invasive similar to

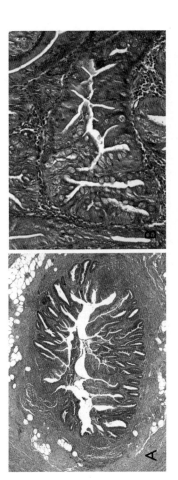

Fig. 6.15 Serrated adenomas circumferentially involve the appendiceal mucosa but, unlike mucinous tumors, they contain goblet and non-goblet epithelial cells with abundant eosinophilic cytoplasm (**a**). The serrated crypts are lined by cells with basally located, pencillate nuclei, similar to those of colorectal serrated adenomas (**b**)

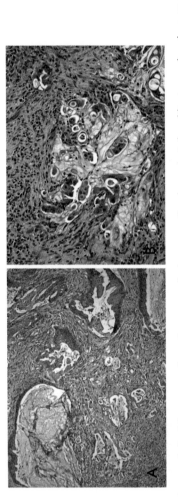

Fig. 6.16 Carcinomas derived from serrated neoplasms may display conventional, or serrated, architecture and copious mucin production (**a**). However, the invasive tumor cells have high-grade cytologic features and are associated with desmoplastic stroma (**b**)

carcinomas, but generally pursue an indolent course, even when metastases are present. Recently, the World Health Organization recommended that such tumors be classified as endocrine, or neuroendocrine, neoplasms, and abandoned the carcinoid terminology, since the biologic behavior of endocrine tumors varies depending on anatomic location and other factors.

Appendiceal endocrine neoplasms display a variety of morphologic features and vary with respect to their biologic potential. Most are comprised of enterochromaffin cells that express serotonin in addition to synaptophysin and chromogranin. These lesions are usually incidentally discovered firm, yellow nodules that occur in the distal tip of the appendix (Fig. 6.17). They contain nests of bland polygonal cells with abundant faintly eosinophilic cytoplasm enmeshed within paucicellular collagenous stroma (Fig. 6.18a). The nuclei are monotonous, smooth, and round, without perceptible atypia, and mitotic figures are lacking (Fig. 6.18b). Endocrine neoplasms derived from L-cells are much less common and express glucagon and peptide YY in addition

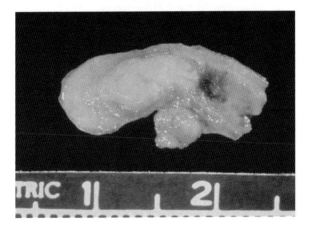

Fig. 6.17 Appendiceal endocrine neoplasms form solid tan-yellow nodules in the distal tip of the appendix

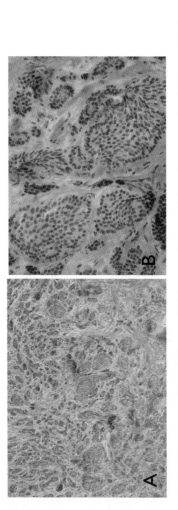

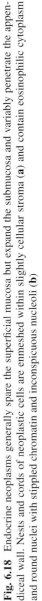

Fig. 6.18 Endocrine neoplasms generally spare the superficial mucosa but expand the submucosa and variably penetrate the appendiceal wall. Nests and cords of neoplastic cells are enmeshed within slightly cellular stroma (**a**) and contain eosinophilic cytoplasm and round nuclei with stippled chromatin and inconspicuous nucleoli (**b**)

to chromogranin and synaptophysin. They also show a predilection for the distal appendix. L-cell endocrine neoplasms contain trabeculae, cords, and, rarely, tubules, of bland endocrine cells with ovoid nuclei and no mitotic activity. Both enterochromaffin and L-cell endocrine neoplasms are generally benign or pursue an indolent clinical course when metastases are present. Tumors that span less than 1 cm are adequately treated by appendectomy, and the risk of metastases from tumors smaller than 2 cm is probably less than 1%. Extensive resection and regional lymph node dissection is reserved for larger tumors, or those associated with metastases, increased mitotic activity, and angioinvasion [1].

Neoplasms that express endocrine markers and contain cytoplasmic mucin have been termed "goblet cell carcinoid tumors", although they are more aggressive than other appendiceal endocrine neoplasms. They do not form nodular masses but, rather, display circumferential growth in the appendiceal submucosa and muscularis propria (Fig. 6.19). Goblet cell carcinoid tumors contain nests and clusters of tumor cells with large mucin vacuoles that

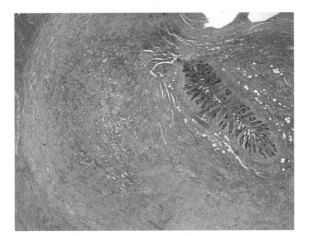

Fig. 6.19 Goblet cell carcinoid tumors spare the mucosa but diffusely infiltrate the appendiceal wall and extend onto the serosal surface

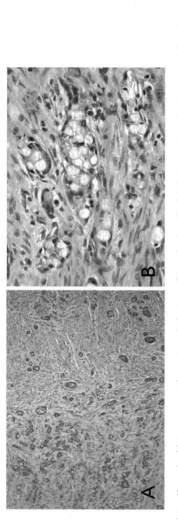

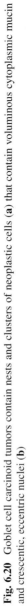

Fig. 6.20 Goblet cell carcinoid tumors contain nests and clusters of neoplastic cells (**a**) that contain voluminous cytoplasmic mucin and crescentic, eccentric nuclei (**b**)

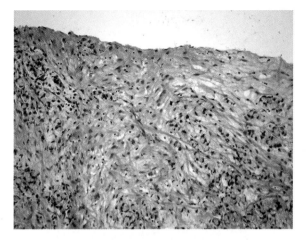

Fig. 6.21 Nests of goblet cell carcinoid tumor diffusely infiltrate peritoneal fat and are associated with a fibroinflammatory tissue response

compress the nuclei (Fig. 6.20). Neoplasms with these features are often of advanced pathologic stage at the time of diagnosis. They penetrate the serosa, occasionally metastasize to regional lymph nodes, and form tumor deposits in the peritoneal cavity and/or ovary, which may prompt frozen section evaluation (Fig. 6.21). Perineural and lymphovascular invasion are frequently observed [13]. In addition, goblet cell carcinoid tumors may precede development of frank adenocarcinomas, which either form glands or resemble signet ring cell or diffuse-type carcinoma, leading some investigators to propose terms, such as "adenocarcinoma ex goblet cell carcinoid" and "mixed goblet cell carcinoid adenocarcinoma" (Fig. 6.22).

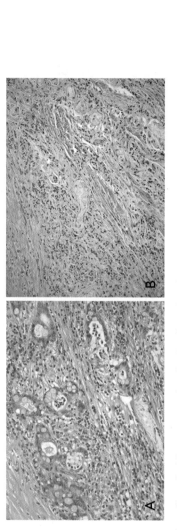

Fig. 6.22 Goblet cell carcinoid tumors occasionally give rise to invasive adenocarcinomas that show glandular differentiation (**a**) or a diffuse growth pattern with signet ring cells (**b**)

References

1. Carr NJ, Sobin LH (2004) Neuroendocrine tumors of the appendix. Semin Diagn Pathol 21(2):108–119
2. Jordan FT, Mazzeo RJ, Hoshal VL (1983) Primary adenocarcinoma of the appendix. Can preoperative or intraoperative diagnosis be made? Am Surg 49(5):278–281
3. Younes M (2005) Frozen section of the gastrointestinal tract, appendix, and peritoneum. Arch Pathol Lab Med 129(12):1558–1564
4. Misdraji J, Young RH (2004) Primary epithelial neoplasms and other epithelial lesions of the appendix (excluding carcinoid tumors). Semin Diagn Pathol 21:120–133
5. Yantiss RK, Shia J, Klimstra DS, Hahn HP, Odze RD, Misdraji J (2009) Prognostic significance of localized extra-appendiceal mucin deposition in appendiceal mucinous neoplasms. Am J Surg Pathol 33(2):248–255
6. Bradley RF, Stewart JH, Russell GB, Levine EA, Geisinger KR (2006) Pseudomyxoma peritonei of appendiceal origin: a clinicopathologic analysis of 101 patients uniformly treated in a single institution, with literature review. Am J Surg Pathol 30(5):551–559
7. Carr NJ, McCarthy WF, Sobin LH (1995) Epithelial noncarcinoid tumors and tumor-like lesions of the appendix: a clinicopathologic study of 184 patients with a multivariate analysis of prognostic factors. Cancer 75(3):757–768
8. Misdraji J, Yantiss RK, Graeme-Cooke FM, Balis UJ, Young RH (2003) Appendiceal mucinous neoplasms: a clinicopathologic analysis of 107 cases. Am J Surg Pathol 27(8):1089–1103
9. Pai RK, Beck AH, Norton JA, Longacre TA (2009) Appendiceal mucinous neoplasms: clinicopathologic study of 116 cases with analysis of factors predicting recurrence. Am J Surg Pathol 33(10):1425–1439
10. Ronnett BM, Zahn CM, Kurman RJ, Kass ME, Sugarbaker PH, Shmookler BM (1995) Disseminated peritoneal adenomucinosis and peritoneal mucinous carcinomatosis: a clinicopathologic analysis of 109 cases with emphasis on distinguishing pathologic features, site of origin, and relationship to "pseudomyxoma peritonei". Am J Surg Pathol 19(12):1390–1408
11. Hamilton SR, Aaltonen LA (1999) Tumours of the appendix. WHO classification of tumours: tumours of the digestive system. WHO Press, Geneva
12. Yantiss RK, Panczykowski A, Misdraji J, Odze RD, Rennert H, Chen Y (2007) A comprehensive study of non-dysplastic and dysplastic serrated polyps of the vermiform appendix. Am J Surg Pathol 31(12):1742–1753
13. Tang LH, Shia J, Soslow RA, et al (2008) Pathologic classification and clinical behavior of the spectrum of goblet cell carcinoid tumors of the appendix. Am J Surg Pathol 32(10):1429–1443

Chapter 7
Frozen Section Evaluation of Anal Disease

Abstract Paget's disease and squamous cell neoplasms are the most common anal disorders to be evaluated by frozen section analysis. Pathologists may be asked to evaluate margin status since their microscopic extent is often greater than is grossly appreciated. Paget's disease may be mimicked by other entities, including reactive squamous cells, koilocytes, and melanocytic proliferations. In situ squamous neoplasms also display features that simulate invasion in frozen sections.

Keywords Paget's disease · Squamous cell neoplasm · Anal intraepithelial neoplasia

Introduction

Lesions of the anal mucosa present unique challenges to the surgeon and pathologist, owing to the tendency for both in situ and invasive neoplasms to display extensive histologic disease, despite their limited gross appearance. The most common diseases subjected to frozen section analysis are Paget's disease and squamous neoplasms, for which evaluation of margin status is important. Unfortunately, a variety of artifacts inherent in frozen sections may complicate interpretation of these cases, as described below.

N.C. Panarelli, R.K. Yantiss, *Frozen Section Library: Appendix,* 113
Colon, and Anus, Frozen Section Library 4, DOI 10.1007/978-1-4419-6584-4_7,
© Springer Science+Business Media, LLC 2010

Paget's Disease

Anal Paget's disease is a malignant neoplasm with a predominantly intraepithelial distribution. The affected area is often eczematous with a flaky, white appearance, resulting from infiltration of the mucosa by malignant mucinous epithelial cells. Anal disease is classified as either primary or secondary Paget's disease. Primary Paget's disease originates from intraepithelial cells derived from apocrine ducts or adnexal stem cells and may be associated with invasive carcinomas of skin adnexae (Fig. 7.1). Secondary Paget's disease reflects the presence of an underlying colonic-type adenocarcinoma of the anorectum with secondary colonization of the squamous mucosa. Management consists of wide local excision for noninvasive disease and abdominoperineal resection with wide excision of the skin for cases associated with underlying carcinoma [1, 2]. Frozen section analysis is often performed to ensure adequate margins.

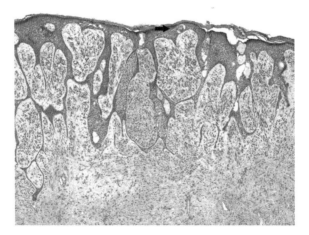

Fig. 7.1 Perianal Paget's disease may reflect the presence of an underlying adenocarcinoma. In this case, the subepithelial connective tissue is expanded by a diffuse-type carcinoma associated with nests of malignant cells (*arrow*) in the overlying mucosa

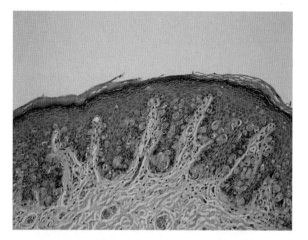

Fig. 7.2 Perianal Paget's disease consists of neoplastic mucinous epithelial cells that populate the squamous mucosa. The cells form nests or linear arrays in the deep mucosa and are variably present in the superficial squamous epithelium

The neoplastic cells of perianal Paget's disease are large and polygonal and contain abundant faintly eosinophilic, or clear, cytoplasm with large atypical nuclei and prominent nucleoli (Fig. 7.2). They are arranged singly or in nests along the basal layer of the squamous epithelium (Fig. 7.3a) but may penetrate the full thickness of the mucosa and display large, hyperchromatic nuclei and mitotic figures (Fig. 7.3b). Assessment of margins by frozen section analysis may be challenging because reactive squamous cells often display perinuclear "halos" that simulate the appearance of neoplastic mucinous cells (Fig. 7.4). However, squamous cells with perinuclear halos are often seen in combination with others that show a lesser degree of clearing, as well as intramucosal edema, and dyskeratotic cells. Isolated neoplastic cells in cases of Paget's disease also resemble melanocytes or intraepithelial Langerhans cells, both of which generally lack substantial cytologic atypia [3] (Fig. 7.5).

When the diagnosis of Paget's disease is not suspected, other entities may be considered in the differential diagnosis. Human

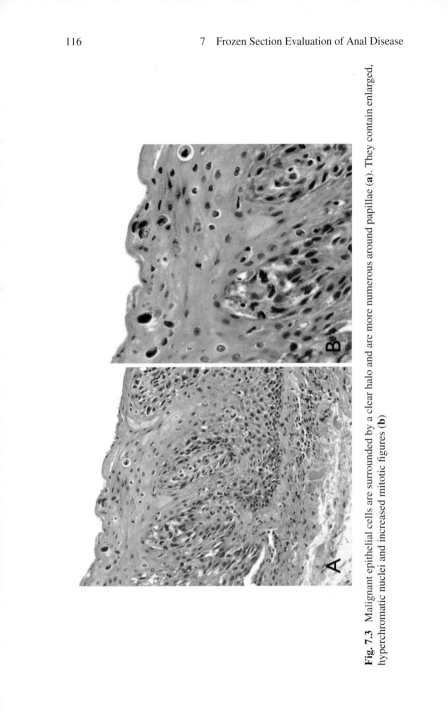

Fig. 7.3 Malignant epithelial cells are surrounded by a clear halo and are more numerous around papillae (**a**). They contain enlarged, hyperchromatic nuclei and increased mitotic figures (**b**)

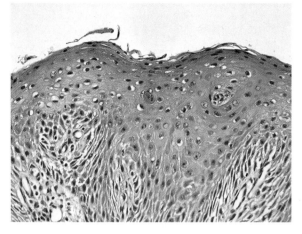

Fig. 7.4 Regenerative changes in squamous epithelial cells adjacent to Paget's disease simulates the appearance of tumor cells, since reactive squamous cells contain perinuclear halos in combination with nuclear enlargement

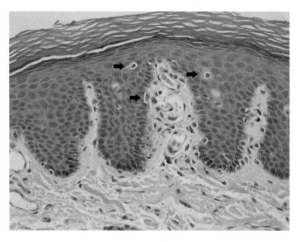

Fig. 7.5 Intra-epithelial Langerhan's cells have abundant faintly eosinophilic cytoplasm and mimic tumor cells of Paget's disease (*arrows*), but lack mitotic activity and do not contain cytoplasmic mucin

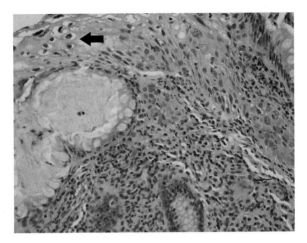

Fig. 7.6 Koilocytosis that results from infection with human papillomavirus may also simulate the appearance of Paget's disease. However, koilocytes lack cytoplasmic mucin and contain crescentic, raisinoid nuclei with hyperchromasia

papillomavirus infection induces koilocytosis, which simulates Paget's disease in frozen sections, although the atypical cells are most numerous in the superficial epithelium and lack mucin (Fig. 7.6). Anal malignant melanomas may also rarely develop. Many of these lesions are partially, or completely, amelanotic and, thus, simulate the clinical appearance of a hemorrhoid or fibroepithelial polyp. Anal melanomas usually grow as solid nests of tumor cells within the subepithelial connective tissue of the anus. However, melanocytes may also infiltrate the squamous mucosa as nests or single cells (Fig. 7.7). Melanocytes are somewhat dyshesive and contain eosinophilic cytoplasm, but they clearly lack mucin and usually have prominent nucleoli.

Squamous Cell Carcinoma

In situ squamous lesions are managed by limited anal mucosal resection, in which case intraoperative frozen section analysis may be used to determine the status of resection margins. Excision

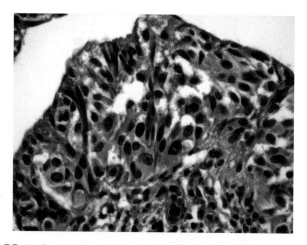

Fig. 7.7 Anal melanoma may involve the squamous or anorectal transitional mucosa. The tumor cells infiltrate as single, or clustered, cells with tapering eosinophilic cytoplasm and large hyperchromatic nuclei. Note the minimal amount of melanin present in this lesion

specimens are usually oriented, in which case the designated margins must be clearly understood before performing frozen section analysis. The deep and lateral margins should be differentially inked and perpendicular sections taken at points closest to the lesion [3]. Chemoradiation is standard first-line therapy for invasive squamous cell carcinoma of the anus, whereas surgical intervention is reserved for patients who develop tumor recurrence following treatment [4]. In this situation, patients undergo abdominoperineal resection with removal of the entire anorectum and frozen sections are usually unnecessary.

Anal intraepithelial neoplasia (AIN) is classified using a three-tiered system (AIN I, AIN II, and AIN III), corresponding to mild, moderate, and severe dysplasia, respectively. Low-grade lesions (AIN I) are treated with local excision or topical agents and generally do not require frozen section analysis. Both AIN II and AIN III are considered to represent high-grade lesions and consist of markedly atypical squamous epithelial cells that populate more than two-thirds of the mucosal thickness (Fig. 7.8). Surgeons may request intraoperative consultations when excising high-grade

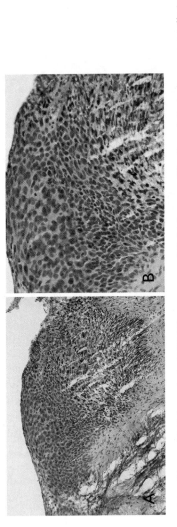

Fig. 7.8 High-grade anal intraepithelial neoplasia (AIN III) appears as a full-thickness proliferation of atypical squamous cells (**a**). The tumor cells contain enlarged, hyperchromatic nuclei and display scattered mitotic figures (**b**)

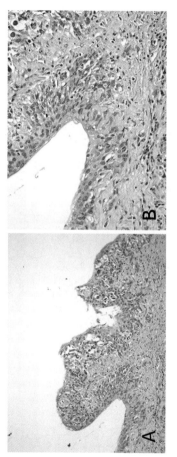

Fig. 7.9 This sample was obtained from an ulcer in an area of high-grade AIN. The epithelium is attenuated, inflamed, and atypical (**a**). The interface between the base of the epithelium and underlying stroma is irregular, simulating the appearance of early invasive carcinoma (**b**)

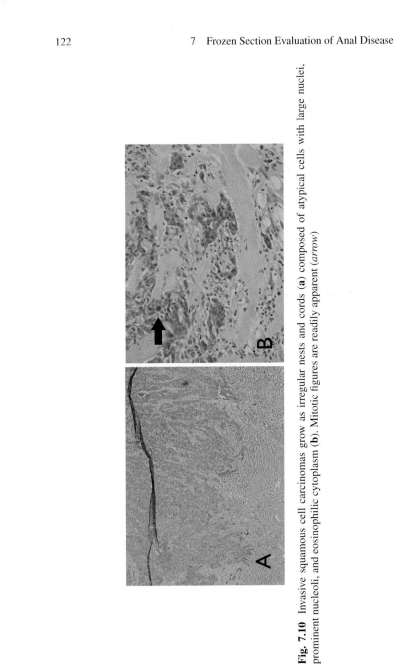

Fig. 7.10 Invasive squamous cell carcinomas grow as irregular nests and cords (**a**) composed of atypical cells with large nuclei, prominent nucleoli, and eosinophilic cytoplasm (**b**). Mitotic figures are readily apparent (*arrow*)

AIN, in order to evaluate the status of the margins or exclude the possibility of invasive carcinoma. Unfortunately, both non-neoplastic squamous epithelium and dysplasia may show features that simulate the appearance of invasive carcinoma, particularly in the setting of superimposed inflammation [3]. The epithelium may be attenuated and contain atypical cells that display an irregular interface with the underlying stroma (Fig. 7.9). Alternatively, AIN may extend down ducts and adnexal structures, mimicking invasive cancer. Therefore, a diagnosis of invasive carcinoma should be reserved for cases in which deep downward extension of individual, or nested, neoplastic cells is present [3] (Fig. 7.10).

References

1. Stacy D, Burrell MO, Franklin EW (1986) Extramammary Paget's disease of the vulva and anus: use of intraoperative frozen-section margins. Am J Obstet Gynecol 155(3):519–523
2. Gaertner WB, Hagerman GF, Goldberg SM, Finne CO (2008) Perianal Paget's disease treated with wide excision and gluteal flap reconstruction: report of a case and review of the literature. Dis Colon Rectum 51(12):1842–1845
3. Longacre TA, Kong CS, Welton ML (2008) Diagnostic problems in anal pathology. Adv Anat Pathol 15:263–278
4. Ryan DP, Mayer RJ (2000) Anal carcinoma: histology, staging, epidemiology, treatment. Curr Opin Oncol 12:345–352

Index

Note: The letters 'f' and 't' following the locators refer to figures and tables respectively.

N.C. Panarelli, R.K. Yantiss, *Frozen Section Library: Appendix, Colon, and Anus*, Frozen Section Library 4, DOI 10.1007/978-1-4419-6584-4, © Springer Science+Business Media, LLC 2010